Praise for Healing Companions

"This book should be required reading for everybody who is considering getting a psychiatric service dog or is working on training them. I really liked its emphasis on choosing the right dog to fit the needs of each person's personality and life. The chapter on assuring that the dog does not become stressed and is treated in an ethical manner is especially helpful. The use of psychiatric service dogs is relatively new compared to other types of service dogs such as guide dogs for the blind, rescue dogs or dogs to help people who use wheel chairs. The combination of both the right dog coupled with positive training methods can further strengthen the human animal bond and help the field of psychiatric service dogs to develop."

—Temple Grandin, author of *Animals in Translation* and *Animals Make us Human*

"Animals are more complete than people. They are wonderful teachers, therapists and role models for us all. Read *Healing Companions* and learn about their ability to guide and heal us all."

—Bernie Siegel, MD, author of *Smudge Bunny*

"Those of us who have seen the miracles that Assistance Dogs perform are still often amazed when we see many of the new tasks that they perform. Assistance dogs pull people in wheel chairs, pick up dropped objects, turn on/off light switches, assist in dressing and undressing and open doors, but they also enhance the socio/emotional life of the handler. Assistance dogs make it possible for a young disabled person to have a friend who is always there, to bridge the social gap when someone ignores or looks the other way. We all know about these benefits, but we are just beginning to learn how highly skilled and loyal assistance dogs serve in other significant ways; for example the psycho-emotional value of an assistance is just beginning to be recognized. In many ways it is just starting, dogs are just beginning to serve, stay tuned."

—Corey Hudson, Chief Executive Officer, Canine Companions for Independence

Healing Companions

Ordinary Dogs and Their Extraordinary Power to Transform Lives

Jane Miller, LISW, CDBC

New Page Books
A Division of The Career Press, Inc.
Franklin Lakes, N.J.

HEALING COMPANIONS
EDITED BY KATE HENCHES
TYPESET BY GINA HOOGERHYDE
Cover design by Lucia Rossman/DigiDog Design
Printed in the U.S.A. by Courier

To order this title, please call toll-free 1-800-CAREER-1 (NJ and Canada: 201-848-0310) to order using VISA or MasterCard, or for further information on books from Career Press.

The Career Press, Inc., 3 Tice Road, PO Box 687,
Franklin Lakes, NJ 07417
www.careerpress.com
www.newpagebooks.com

Library of Congress Cataloging-in-Publication Data

CIP data available upon request.

Dedication

This book is dedicated to Umaya. She was the catalyst and inspiration in discovering my life's work and passion. This book is a tribute to Umaya and all the dogs that have changed our lives with unconditional love and commitment. Thanks, Umaya, for leading the way.

A portion of the proceeds from this book will be donated to the "Umaya Fund," which was established to help cover the costs of healthcare for assistance dogs for those without financial resources at Lakewood Animal Hospital in Lakewood, Ohio. Donations to the Umaya fund may be sent to:

Lakewood Animal Hospital
ATTN: The Umaya Fund
14587 Madison Ave.
Lakewood, Ohio 44107

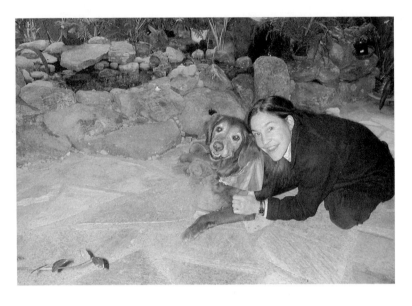

Umaya, who started the healing journey, shares a peaceful moment with Jane in their private oasis. This book is dedicated to Umaya; her stoicism, wisdom, and gentle loving spirit touched so many lives that can live on through her legacy in this book.

Acknowledgments

This book would not exist if Umaya and I had not been blessed by the extraordinary healthcare professionals that saved both of our lives. We are both indebted to the loving, knowledgeable, caring support we received from Robert Barney, DVM, Neal Sivula, DVM, Allen Schoen, DVM, MS, and Victor Fazio, MD (The Cleveland Clinic Foundation). They not only provided exceptional care, but assisted Umaya and me in exploring complementary modalities of healing to maximize quality of life. I am grateful to Dr. Fazio for believing in my resilience and stoicism, and providing me with the opportunity to learn to enjoy each and every moment.

This book has been a dream of mine for years. It has been a long journey filled with sadness and joy, but most of all an accomplishment filled with the love, support, and generous caring of so many. I owe this book to all of the contributors who shared their personal stories so freely. I am also grateful to Gloria Gilbert Stoga, President of Puppies Behind Bars, for her support, feedback, and commitment to improving the lives of our wounded warriors with PTSD. At NEADS, Sheila O'Brien, former CEO, and John Moon, Chief Communications Officer, were always available to provide suggestions, feedback, and resources. Micky Niego provided the wisdom of her years of working in the field as well as knowledge, insights, and tremendous support throughout this process.

I am indebted to Alan Beck (Purdue University, School of Veterinary Medicine, Director, Center of The Human Animal Bond), Toni Eames (IAADP Board member and Treasurer), and Ed Eames (IAADP Board member and President), Corey Hudson, (Chief Executive Officer, Canine Companions for Independence), and Dr. Stephen Porges, PhD (Univ. Of Illinois, Director Brain-Body Center) for discussing their research and providing their knowledge in this field to enhance the accuracy of the information presented in this book.

I would like to acknowledge as well Joan Froling, IAADP, Chairperson and Editor of *Partners Forum* for her dedication, commitment, generosity, and meticulous reading of the manuscript. She shared her experience, wisdom, and expertise in the field of assistance dogs, and went over and above in providing feedback and input. Joan is a renowned authority in the assistance dog field, and I am honored that she agreed to write the Foreword and provided the extremely useful task lists included in the appendix of the book.

Thanks to Mary Basu, photographer extraordinaire (see *www.furinfocus.com*) for formatting the photos and capturing the beautiful bonds between a contributor and her PSDs and the author's headshot with her two co-therapists. With deepest gratitude to Tim Paxton at The Copyshop, Oberlin, Ohio, for his help in formatting the manuscript.

I am deeply appreciative of the endorsements provided by Bonnie Bergin, Temple Grandin, Corey Hudson, Belleruth Naparstek, Allen Schoen, and Bernie Siegel.

They say "it takes a village," and I discovered that as I wrote this book the support of friends, family, and individuals I barely knew exceeded my expectations. Bob Miller, my brother, and Jennifer Josephy, my stepmother, graciously provided me with professional guidance about publishing throughout this process. My mother instilled in me from a young age the importance and value of standing up for what you believe in. She modeled for me the value of activism and power of education, both of which contributed to my motivation for writing this book. I would also like to acknowledge my dear friend of more than 20 years, Kerry Langan. A fellow author and editor of a number of anthologies, Kerry generously devoted her time to reading and rereading every chapter even while writing her own book.

Words can't adequately express the depths of gratitude to my agent, Deirdre Mullane, who believed in this book and my deep commitment to educate others about the healing power of dogs from the first day we spoke. She worked day and night with me on this book, always available and willing to provide her wisdom, feedback, and knowledge without hesitation. All of the staff at New Page Books have been steadfastly supportive and wonderful to work with.

Writing these acknowledgements is like accepting an Oscar, with not enough time to thank everyone before the music starts playing. To anyone I have failed to specifically acknowledge, know that in my heart I cherish the tremendous support, love, respect, generosity, and caring I have felt from one and all. I am honored to have known so many special two-legged and four-legged (and finned, winged, and so on) creatures, and am especially grateful to all the dogs that have shared my life from childhood to the present, especially Simcha and Ahava, who remained constantly by my side as I wrote this book. (I hope my cat Toby forgives me.) With deepest gratitude to all of those who helped make this book a reality.

Contents

Foreword

When I grew up in the 1950s, guide dogs for the blind were a familiar sight and very much admired. Many years later, I was intrigued to learn of a few programs looking into whether or not a dog could offer something more than companionship to individuals with a disability other than blindness.

As a professional dog trainer who had developed mobility limitations, I was fortunate in 1990 to come across a pioneering organization in Michigan that was training hearing dogs for the deaf and service dogs for persons with disabilities other than blindness or deafness. Paws With A Cause helped me to train my 20-month-old Samoyed to assist me to get through heavy commercial doors in a wheelchair, bring in the groceries, fetch a portable phone in a crisis, and perform other useful tasks that enabled me to greatly reduce my dependency on family members, lessen pain and fatigue, and eventually to live and travel on my own. The resulting tremendous improvement in quality of life was so uplifting, it inspired me to become deeply involved with the assistance dog movement at the local, national and international level in the years that followed.

I'm probably best known as cofounder and chairperson of the International Association of Assistance Dog Partners. IAADP is a non profit "self-help" organization which has enabled disabled persons partnered with guide, hearing, and service dogs to work together since 1993 to foster the assistance dog movement through a global networking publication, Website, many advocacy and education campaigns, peer support initiatives, and 14 conferences held in conjunction with Assistance Dogs Internationals conference in the United States, Canada, and the United Kingdom. IAADP has grown from a small group to more than 2,500 Partner members in the last 16 years.

I also have volunteered my skills as a professional dog trainer since 1996 to Sterling Service Dogs, a program that does conventional placements and gives lessons to disabled students who live within driving distance, providing they have a suitable dog to train as a service dog to assist them with mobility and/ or a psychiatric disability.

IAADP has received thousands of queries over the years from individuals who are struggling with mentally disabling conditions like severe depression, panic disorder, or post-traumatic stress disorder. Most get in touch after reading the article I published on IAADP's Website in 2001, "Service Dog Tasks for Psychiatric Disabilities." They want to know how they can obtain a well-mannered service dog who will reliably perform the requested tasks whenever needed in the workplace, a school classroom, on a bus, or on the subway? Regretfully, it has been difficult to find programs with high standards that specialize in this kind of placement in most states. Because the majority will have to investigate other options for the acquisition and training of a suitable dog, I was very interested to learn of Jane Miller's book, *Healing Companions*.

This is the first book I've read that is devoted to the subject of service dogs for men and women who face the hardships of living with a chronic mental illness. It is the first to offer guidance to such individuals, to their families, and to mental healthcare professionals in the effort to increase their chances of achieving a successful outcome and to help them to avoid certain pitfalls if they decide to go down this road. Impressive in scope and easy to read due to Jane's unpretentious writing style, there is much to commend as the reader learns how a task trained dog, commonly termed a "psychiatric service dog," can become a valuable adjunct to conventional therapy.

Jane introduces the reader to men and women who have been battling different kinds of chronic mental illness and their service dogs who help them cope and function. Through their stories, the reader will learn about different aspects of the lifestyle choice we call "assistance dog partnership," beginning with ways that partnership with a task trained service dog can empower a handler to cope much more effectively with certain symptoms or with situations that trigger hypervigilance, a panic attack, or dissociative episodes.

Something that added considerable interest to the book for me were task ideas I had not come across before, a couple of which I plan to share with my students. Jane is an innovative trainer and one willing to invest months of time in achieving the desired outcome. Hopefully some examples given herein will lead to other partners and/or therapists identifying a problem and then finding a clever trainer who can come up with a way the dog can accomplish the goal, something firmly grounded in both a dog's capabilities and limitations.

Jane also includes interviews with military veterans who have post traumatic stress disorder. Their stories illuminate how working with a service dog could improve someone's capacity to handle the debilitating effects of that mental injury. A service dog is not a change to a universal panacea, but for some individuals such as those included here, there can be no doubt this has proven to be an important coping mechanism.

Jane does not soft-pedal the issues that can arise, such as the cost of vet bills and family tensions, or the fact the first dog you select may not be happy in this career. She discusses ethical issues every handler should be aware of, and the question of retirement and a successor dog. There is also a treasure trove of referrals to other books and Website articles on a number of the topics covered in each chapter, enabling readers to further educate themselves on areas of particular concern or interest. It is a thought-provoking book and one that has much to offer anyone considering training their own service dog. It would also be a great addition to the library of any trainer or healthcare professional, so they can help clients "to look before they leap."

This is a book that is long overdue. It encourages a serious, responsible approach to incorporating a service dog into the life of someone disabled by a mental illness. It also verifies that many dogs are capable of providing extraordinary benefits if given the special training and love that a service dog needs to excel.

—Joan Froling

Introduction: How the Healing Journey Began

Several years ago I discovered something powerful about the dogs who share many of our lives. Though all dogs provide love, comfort, joy, and support, for some people, dogs actually have the ability to transform lives. Although I have been in clinical practice as a therapist for years, this isn't something I learned through professional training. The catalyst was a tiny furball named Umaya who came home with me on Christmas Eve. Here's how our journey began.

After a dozen years of working and attending graduate school, I finally moved into my own house in October 1992. My first priority was to get a dog; furniture could wait. As a child of divorce, I recalled that the most memorable, life-altering gift my father ever gave us was a black Labrador Retriever pup we named Tasha. As I grew up, she was my best friend and confidante, especially while going through the trials and tribulations of adolescence. Tasha taught me how extraordinary the bond between a human and animal can be, and I always knew that once I had a home of my own I wanted to find another Tasha. However, I also knew if I adopted another black Lab, she might remind me too much of Tasha's absence, and eventually I fell in love with a breed with a similar disposition the beautiful dark Golden Retrievers.

When I started to look for my new dog, I discovered a breeder of Goldens less than 5 miles away from my home. At our first meeting, I was greeted by a boy aged about 17 years who lived with his family on the farm where they raised the dogs. As a child, he had suffered a serious accident when the combine he was riding went up in flames, and, although he had survived, he still bore the scars of his accident, despite numerous plastic surgeries and skin grafts. As we walked out into the yard to meet the dogs, he told me how he started breeding dark Golden Retrievers after the accident, and he credited the dogs for giving him back his life. The dogs accepted him completely for who he was, not what he looked like. I was so touched by his story, and seeing how deeply the dogs loved him, I knew I'd find my pup here. The next litter was due October 30th. I could hardly wait.

When the day finally came for me to meet the litter, the first pup I picked up curled happily into my lap. But after a few moments she got frisky, and when I put her down she immediately peed. I knew at that moment she was the one because she wouldn't pee on me! We painted her toenails purple so we would know she was mine, and I named her Umaya, which means stability. Then, a few weeks after Umaya entered my life, I received her AKC papers to discover that her dam's name was Tasha!

I brought my darling pup home on Christmas Eve, and, once I let her out of my arms, Umaya scampered about the house, sniffing here and there with her mouth full of toys, investigating everything but with her eyes glued always on me. She slept with me from the first day, cuddled with me, and taught me how to play. From the start it seemed as though we communicated even without words—she seemed to know what I was thinking and feeling—and my friends remarked that she seemed to embody one of my favorite sayings: "Every day is a gift." Looking at that lively puppy, I could not have foreseen where this relationship would take us during the next 12 years, nor the enormous impact she would have on my work. Who could have guessed that she would not only change my life but that of my clients as well?

Umaya went everywhere with me, and my days happily revolved around her needs. Within a week of her homecoming, however, I spotted blood on her blanket. I immediately took her to the veterinarian, who diagnosed a urinary tract infection. Though the breeder offered to replace her, I wouldn't hear of it. Umaya and I had bonded. We'd get through her illness together, as we would the many other problems that we would share during the course of our loving and joyful relationship. When I was unable to attend my grandmother's funeral because of a blizzard, I listened to the service over the telephone. Umaya, still a puppy, crawled onto my lap and licked my tears away, and, when the service was over and I'd hung up, she brought me a toy to play with. Umaya always knew what I needed and she never failed to bring a smile to my face.

But there were bigger troubles ahead. When Umaya was 5, I discovered a lump one day on her left hip while I was giving her a massage. When I brought her to the vet, he diagnosed her with fibrosarcoma, a skin cancer not commonly seen in dogs, and he recommended radiation treatment as a precaution to prevent the disease from spreading. Without treatment, her likelihood of survival was quite slim. Because the veterinary hospital was close to my office, during her 18 days of treatment I started to bring Umaya to work with me. From the first day, Umaya walked into the waiting room and began to make the rounds of clients, greeting each one with a mouth full of toys and her happy smile. Without ever making a complaint or a whine, she continued to find joy in every day, every little wonder to wag about.

Umaya successfully completed her treatment and seemed well on the path to recovery when, a few weeks later while she and I were taking a walk, two dogs flew out of a neighbor's garage and raced to attack her. Though Umaya turned away from them in an attempt to ward off the attack by appearing submissive, the dogs latched onto her side near her back left leg, close to where the tumor had been. There was blood everywhere.

Terrified, I brought Umaya home, and within half an hour she was in the hospital. Two hours of surgery followed. Fortunately, the attack had missed all of her major organs. The fact that she was on antibiotics to prevent infections during her radiation therapy gave Umaya an edge. Fearing that Umaya would be overstressed if she spent yet another night in the hospital, her veterinarian sent her home with me, along with antiobiotics and a list of signs to look for during the night. When Umaya awoke near me the next morning, after having survived the attack and ensuing surgery, I knew that she would live.

Following the attack, although Umaya displayed behaviors indicating that she may have been suffering from stress, she continued to go to work with me, hopping on three legs and bright with the glow of being alive. But from that period on, perhaps because of adhesions or the buildup of scar tissue, Umaya lost the ability to use her rear legs until she received acupuncture, which helped decrease the inflammation and gave her back the ability to ambulate. At the same time, I was recovering from surgery of my own after an exhaustive (and unfortunately unnecessary) operation years earlier to locate the source of internal bleeding. I struggled with chronic pain and I could not have been more sympathetic to Umaya's plight. She and I seemed to be leading somewhat parallel lives and both benefited from acupuncture treatments.

During all of this time, Umaya continued to accompany me to work, and for me the therapeutic process was transformed. She began to attend therapy sessions, lying in a corner of the room while the clients talked. She became a mirror image of my clients' feelings, helping them become more in tune with their own emotions. If they were sad, she'd walk over to them and look pouty; if they were angry she'd chew her rubber bones voraciously, or she'd bring her toy over in an attempt to diffuse their anger. Frequently, clients would begin petting Umaya, start talking, and not even realize that they were sharing painful memories, releasing old hurts, and freeing their spirits. Umaya wordlessly provided support and a sense of calm. As I saw clients experiencing Umaya's presence in such a profound way, I began to consider how powerful it would be for some of them to have a dog of their own.

In our fast-paced world, doctors are often quick to advise patients suffering from traumatic stress, depression, anxiety, and other emotional and psychological problems that their ills can be solved through the use of one medication or another. Too many people think the pill itself is a "magic bullet" that will make their lives happier, easier, and more secure. It isn't. Medications must be taken under careful supervision, and many anti-depressant drugs carry the risk of negative side effects, including in extreme cases suicidal tendencies. Although many individuals do require medication, which has helped countless people, there are other pill-free choices that are extremely beneficial and may not have been considered. For many people one choice that they may have never heard of, either by itself or in combination with drug therapy and psychotherapy, might make all the difference.

Service dogs have been assisting the blind, the hearing-impaired, and those in wheelchairs and with other disabilities for a long time. There are also Therapy dogs who help enhance quality of life for many people by visiting hospitals, nursing homes, and, other institutions providing comfort and support. Umaya's strength and calming influence were a revelation to me, and when I saw the way that my clients responded to her, I began to realize that having a dog could have a profound impact on some of my clients' lives.

This is not just the story of our journey, however; it's a window onto the world of psychiatric service dogs for people with invisible disabilities, showing how the dogs can change and enhance the lives of their human companions. In the following chapters, we'll meet some of these amazing dogs and see how they have helped a number of individuals improve their lives in profound and unexpected ways, allowing them to gain self-esteem, self-confidence, assertiveness, and so much more. These dogs provide emotional support, as all dogs do, but they are specifically trained to perform certain tasks unique to the individual's needs. Through the stories of these dogs, I hope to show how you, a friend, or a family member how he or she might benefit from such a healing companion.

In addition to these remarkable stories, this book will also explain which dogs are the right candidates for the job, which dogs are not, and how to tell the difference. Here's a hint: It has nothing to do with the dog's breed. Mixed-breed dogs are very well suited to assist those with invisible disabilities. These dogs can be in-home companions or full-time Service dogs who also accompany their companions out in public and to work. I'll discuss how these dogs are trained, how the dog may impact other members of the family, and how to make life more comfortable and less stressful for the dogs while they are undertaking their essential tasks. I'll also provide a helpful list of resources for further information, support, and services.

For anyone who may not know about the profound benefits that these service dogs may bring, as well as for anyone who loves dogs and enjoys learning more about their value to their companions, I hope this book will serve as an informative, practical, and inspirational guide.

Umaya started me on this extraordinary path. Now, share the journey of my clients and others who have opened their hearts to a service dog and found a healing beyond their expectations.

1

Mindy's Story: Umaya Leads the Way

There's something calming about the presence of a dog.

When I began to bring Umaya to my office, she spread joy wherever she went, but when she walked among my clients, her tail wagging so hard that her entire rear end wiggled in turn, it was just about impossible to ignore her enthusiasm. She would move from person to person in the waiting room, inviting them to play. The clients simply loved her, but Umaya would ultimately prove capable of so much more. There was no design behind my discovery of Umaya's gift. It was, you might say, serendipitous.

For some time I had been working with a young woman named Mindy, who was in her 20s but looked younger. An incest survivor, Mindy had lived a life of which nightmares are made. Violent crimes always leave the survivor feeling insecure, but imagine what it must be like when the violence begins in infancy. Experiencing night after night of sexual abuse, Mindy never felt safe even in her own room. Although it is often a male relative who carries out the abuse, that wasn't the case here. Mindy's abusers were her mother and her sister. A mother is normally equated with nurturing, safety, protection, and love, but the unthinkable had happened to Mindy as a child.

It came as no surprise that Umaya was a gentle support during Mindy's sessions. People often feel comfortable and safe with a dog and will talk in its presence when they are uncomfortable talking with another person. As Mindy opened up and began to reveal her childhood horrors, her stress level would naturally increase. And there would be Umaya, rapidly rubbing her tongue on the rug in response to the tension in the room, as if she were trying to get a bad taste out of her mouth. Mindy would look at Umaya and realize that Umaya was reflecting her own stress, that she was mirroring the uncomfortable feelings Mindy was releasing as a result of describing her trauma when she, herself, didn't know how to deal with those emotions. But what happened next with Mindy and Umaya was even more extraordinary.

One day, I walked into my office for a session to find Mindy waiting, talking to Umaya. But her voice sounded different. Childlike. As I observed her interacting with Umaya, I realized that Mindy wasn't acting "like Mindy," but had assumed another personality. I understood then that Mindy had multiple personality disorder, the result of the trauma she had experienced as a child. Umaya had not just brought out a childlike quality in Mindy; she had coaxed out a child, another self, within her.

When children are abused in infancy, before the personality has had a chance to form, multiple personalities may be created to help the child cope with extremely difficult circumstances. In therapy, the multiples can look to the therapist as a comforting figure, a parent, but Mindy was convinced that they saw Umaya in that role. The little ones, as Mindy referred to those parts, wanted Umaya to protect them, "almost like they wanted to be enveloped in her love."

Though there was nothing unusual about her outward appearance, before Mindy realized that she was a multiple, she felt like she was living in the midst of a war zone. As Mindy and I continued to work together, we would ultimately discover that she had several parts within her that had helped her survive: some male, some female, some adults, some children, sometimes aligning themselves with each other in groups. As Mindy began to remember her difficult past, while working with a psychiatrist as well as with me, the memories were disturbing, and she never knew what would set her off. She was balancing three jobs to make enough money to survive, and she felt as if she was constantly running, like "the lid on everything had flown off." Every act became a chore and Mindy had to relearn basic life skills, to feed herself, to bathe herself, to take care of herself. She had to learn to be more direct and assertive with others. And she needed to find a sense of security, of love.

During this difficult time, it seemed that Mindy was less afraid of dogs than of humans. Whereas dogs make their needs known simply and directly, Mindy's experience with people up until that point was that they communicated through a series of mixed messages so she couldn't make sense of anything. When her psychiatrist and I both suggested that she should consider adopting a dog, Mindy looked at me one day and said, "I need an Umaya."

Many discussions ensued about this prospect. Mindy wanted to know what was involved in caring for a dog, and how much responsibility she would be assuming if she adopted a canine companion. She wanted to understand what the dog would need in order to have a good life, and she needed to believe that she could take care of those needs. And we had concerns as well. Because Mindy has multiple personalities, we had to consider what would happen if any of the parts didn't like a dog or became jealous of the time Mindy spent with her companion. Then there were the daily walks, playtime, and training to consider. She would have to feed and groom a dog, as well as take it regularly to the veterinarian. She would have to be responsible for another life.

Mindy's landlord didn't allow dogs, and Mindy didn't think she was capable of asking for special permission because, as a childhood abuse survivor, she felt intensely worthless. After Mindy's psychiatrist wrote a "prescription" for a dog, Mindy was finally able to approach her landlord, but it would take another couple of months before she would bring a dog home. When Mindy underwent a brief hospitalization, she understandably had mixed emotions about going forward with our plan. The thought of getting a dog helped her to recover and leave the hospital, but she worried about being able to take care of herself and about bringing a dog home into her environment. Mindy had always been so careful not to burden anyone else with her problems that she found it hard to get close to another human being. But Mindy's doctor and I were convinced that the dog would be a lifeline for her.

Once she had committed to the idea, Mindy was adamant about getting a shelter dog, and she and I visited the shelter numerous times together. We made several trips as Mindy got to know the dogs, until one day she spotted a black and tan Terrier/Beagle mix who seemingly held no appeal for anyone until Mindy came along. The dog's beautiful, soulful eyes and her absurdly barrel-chested body captivated Mindy immediately, and the feeling was mutual. After she and I convinced the shelter employee, who expressed some concern about letting a dog go home with a young woman who had just been released from a psychiatric ward, Mindy received approval to adopt her dog. Mindy knew that the little Terrier/Beagle cross, whom she named Ninna, was meant to be hers.

The name Ninna had special significance for Mindy. While being sexually assaulted by her mother and sister, Mindy would disassociate from the act, her mind floating free, carrying her away to the home of a sea hag named Ninna who lived on the beach. "She changed form every time we visited her," Mindy recalls, remembering that Ninna would take them—her parts—on night flights "above the ocean and through the stars." Ninna became their caretaker and protector in the fantasy world that the young Mindy and her parts created, someone who cared about them, protected them, and taught them how to survive. The canine Ninna became for Mindy the real-life embodiment of that personality: the caretaker and protector.

As Mindy assumed the responsibility for the care and feeding of her dog, she learned to begin to care for herself as well. Before Ninna, Mindy had spent so much time disassociating while there was constant chatter in her head that she couldn't focus or function. Now, when she put her hand on Ninna, Mindy had to remind herself that she was in her own apartment, her own bedroom, where no one could hurt her anymore. "She helped us rediscover how to be present," Mindy relates. And with Ninna in her life, Mindy has learned to establish regular habits—eating, bathing, going to work—and Mindy loves the long walks that she and Ninna share. Ninna has helped Mindy discover "the beauty and magic in the every day rituals and looking forward to small things every day." When out on walks together if they passed someone that made Mindy feel uncomfortable or stressed Ninna would block the intruder from coming too close to Mindy.

To many who don't know Mindy well, her life appears normal. She has graduated from college and she now holds a responsible job. She has had the occasional set back, but her concern for Ninna helps her through difficult times. The routine established between Mindy and Ninna has helped Mindy with the basic activities of daily living. If Mindy forgets to feed Ninna, Ninna will nudge and pester Mindy, reminding Mindy to feed her, which reminds Mindy to feed herself. Mindy knows that Ninna needs her to be healthy enough to care for her, ensuring that Mindy takes care of herself as well and reinforcing her need to stay on her medication. In addition to providing Mindy with a feeling of stability and security, Ninna has been trained in specific tasks that help to mitigate the effects of Mindy's disability. When Mindy is crying or upset, Ninna disrupts the emotional upheaval Mindy is experiencing by nudging, pawing, and licking her, and this physical stimulation diverts Mindy's attention, helps her regain a sense of calm, and can prevent her from entering a disassociative state.

There have been unique challenges. Not all of Mindy's personalities wanted a dog, and when one of the parts wanted to kick Ninna, Mindy had to physically remove herself from the room in order to ensure that that part didn't harm her. Mindy was able to manage these feelings, but this concern was a serious reminder to Mindy that she needed someone else in place, a backup, to look out for the dog's safety if she were hospitalized or had some problem dealing with the dog or meeting the dog's needs. But Mindy knew that I would be there for her if she and Ninna needed help. Love, security, and a sense of stability walked into Mindy's life and heart the day she brought

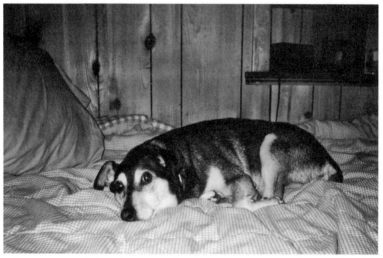

Even at rest, Ninna's eyes and calm presence provide Mindy with reassurance and a sense of security.

Ninna home. Now, when Mindy goes to sleep at night touching Ninna, she feels safe.

Both Mindy and Ninna approach life somewhat warily. "She's great! But she can be very demanding," says Mindy of her canine companion. Fortunately, Ninna doesn't bark a lot, which is good, because some of Mindy's parts who are children are scared by barking. They are also scared of sudden movements, as is Ninna, who often twitches first when Mindy reaches to pet her. Mindy has learned to read Ninna's body language and understand when she needs to be removed from a particular situation. She knows that having a dog means taking responsibility for protecting the dog as well as loving and nurturing her. They're two survivors helping each other.

Somehow, it seems preordained that Mindy and Ninna would come together. "When I see her sprawled out in a very elegant, absurdly relaxed pose and she gives me that look over her shoulder, like, 'Oh! It's you! You're home!' I think, 'Wow! I did something great! She is so comfortable. It's fantastic!'" Mindy and her parts are also finally learning to be comfortable both within a space and within themselves. For Mindy, seeing Ninna like that is similar to a gentle elbow nudge saying that she can try it, too, that it's okay to relax in her own home. "It's amazing to love and be loved back, and to be able to take it for granted sometimes, to never question it, it's always there. And I don't think we've ever had that before," says Mindy, as if she is speaking for Ninna as well. Together they have forged a relationship filled with unconditional love.

As Mindy looks to the future, she's concerned about how long she and Ninna have together, or if she could live without a dog again. She knows that every moment is precious. When the time comes, Mindy will honor Ninna by choosing another canine companion with whom she can share her life, a fitting tribute to this special dog.

As Mindy's story reveals, having a dog to love and care for can have a profound and beneficial effect on the lives of those with emotional challenges. We are accustomed to thinking about the usefulness of a guide dog for the blind or a service dog to assist someone in a wheelchair. We are less familiar with the idea of a healing companion for individuals who are suffering from emotional challenges, such as depression, anxiety, post-traumatic stress, or other invisible disabilities. For those who are coping with these challenges, a PSD may be a critical part of their recovery and a source of much needed comfort, responsibility, and assistance.

However, PSDs are not for everyone. Every individual has different needs, desires, and capabilities, and you should explore all of your options to determine the right course regarding finding a suitable dog and how to integrate the dog into your life. In the chapters that follow, we'll look more closely at how individuals who experience agoraphobia, panic attacks, depression, bipolar disorder, traumatic stress, eating disorders, and other mental health challenges have benefited from bringing a PSD home. We'll also look at the legal protections and practical considerations you might face. But first, here are some basic questions to consider before embarking on this journey with your own healing companion:

1. Are you legally disabled? A PSD is not simply a welcome canine companion but a service dog trained in very specific ways to mitigate the effects of the disabilities of its handler. In order to qualify as disabled under the Americans with Disabilities Act (ADA), your emotional or psychiatric condition must "substantially limit one or more major life activities" such as caring for oneself, speaking, breathing, concentrating, thinking, eating, communicating, sleeping, and working. Further, you must "be regarded as having" and there "must be a record of" your having such an impairment. For you to enjoy all of the legal protections afforded to you under this act, you must fit the definition of disabled, and your dog must be individually and specifically trained in work or tasks that mitigate the effects of your disability. (For the full text of the ADA, see *www. ada.gov/pubs/adastatute08.htm.*)

2. Do you have the resources financially to care for a dog? Consider realistically whether you can assume the burden of feeding and sheltering a dog. In addition to the cost of food, kennel supplies, and toys, keep in mind that you will need to have regular veterinary visits and will need to consider some professional training. You must be willing to make an investment in the health and well-being of your dog over the course of its lifetime.

3. Do you have the time and temperament to care for a dog? Dogs require daily attention, walks, feeding, grooming, and love. If you have had a dog in the past, you may already feel certain that you can assume these responsibilities capably. If not, consider carefully the

impact that taking care of the dog will have on your schedule and lifestyle.

4. Do you have a network of people supporting the integration of a PSD into your life? Anyone with a dog knows that sometimes you need help, someone to assist you taking the dog to the vet or with the occasional walk or trip to the dog run. For people coping with emotional difficulties, there may be numerous instances when you are temporarily unable to care for your dog. You will need to make sure that there are a number of reliable people to whom you can turn if such a situation arises.

5. Does your family support your choice? Bringing a new dog into the home means changes for everyone. Consider how your bond with the dog will affect the feelings of other members of your family. Make sure that they understand the dog's therapeutic role, and be clear about how responsibilities for the dog will be handled.

6. Do you have a therapist who supports your choice to get a dog? Talk with your regular therapist about the benefits of having the dog in your life, what outcome you expect, and what role he or she will have in helping you gain the full benefit from your dog. Many professionals may not yet be familiar with the growing role of PSDs, but you will benefit if your therapist is open and encouraging as you begin your own journey with your PSD.

7. Are you willing to work with a professional trainer to train your dog to realize its full potential as a PSD? In this book, we will discuss how PSDs are trained and the tasks they can perform. However, there will be instances

when you will need to work with a professional trainer who can help both you and the dog learn to mitigate the effects of your disability, interact well together, and behave appropriately in public.

8. Can you deal with the sometimes-unwanted attention that a PSD will bring when you are out in public? Dogs frequently attract strangers, welcoming their advances and delighting in the attention. A PSD may also invite curious glances or comments from others who may want to know more about the dog's abilities and training. Consider whether you will find such attention an opportunity to interact with others or a painful or awkward burden.

9. Are you prepared to cope with the dog's need to retire, deciding the dog is not the right fit, or the dog's aging and death? Inevitably, there will come a time when your PSD is no longer able to be an active part of your therapy, and this transition can be painful. Consider whether you will be able to withstand these normal feelings while providing the care your dog deserves after a lifetime of service.

Despite these concerns, for many individuals a dog can be a remarkable aid to a fuller, more productive life. As Mindy remembers the many years that she and Ninna worked together, she recalls appreciatively, "Ninna not only helped me feel safe in the world, but she got me out into it to discover all that surrounded me. She made the world navigable." Read on to discover how others learned to navigate their way through life with the extraordinary benefit of a healing companion.

2

Canine Rx: Finding the Right Companion

In recent years, the benefits of psychiatric service dogs to their handlers have been the subject of much media attention, from television news and advocate blogs to the pages of *The New York Times*, *The Wall Street Journal*, and *The New Yorker*. Yet for many people, the concept is still new and there are lots of questions. What is a psychiatric service dog (PSD)? Am I eligible for a PSD? Where do I get one? How do I train it? Which kinds of dogs are best suited to the task?

As with many initiatives that have transformed the daily lives of disabled Americans, the introduction of psychiatric service dogs stemmed from the passage of the Americans with Disabilities Act by Congress in 1990. Along with curb-cut sidewalks, wider store aisles, and obstacle-free building entryways, the ADA provided broader protections for service animals beyond their utilization as guide dogs for the blind, which had begun around the end of World War I. The 1990 act was built on the foundation of the Rehabilitation Act of 1973, which prohibited discrimination on the basis of disability in any program run or funded by the federal government. In 1990, the ADA expanded coverage to a broader group of disabled individuals, so that anyone with "a physical or mental impairment that substantially limits one or more of the major life activities…is entitled to certain protections under the law against discrimination in employment, housing, transportation, and other areas of public life." There are ongoing legal challenges and reinterpretations of the ADA, but with its broader legal protections, the act opened the door to a greater role for service dogs in assisting those with invisible disabilities. (For the current accepted definitions and interpretations of the ADA, see Appendix 3 and Resource pages 235-236.) Now, we are beginning to see that dogs can significantly aid not only individuals who are deaf or blind, but also those who are suffering from panic disorder, post-traumatic stress disorder, depression, agoraphobia, bipolar disorder, and other emotional ills.

As a trusted companion, the psychiatric service dog is literally a bridge between the handler and his or her environment. The complex tasks and routines practiced by the dog provide a level of independence and can advance the handler's attempts to leave "familiar territory," be it home, neighborhood, or family, break ritualistic behavior patterns or "try on" entry-level social skills. Depending on the individual's disability, PSDs have been trained to guide a handler disoriented by anxiety, conduct a room search to alleviate fear of intruders or the unknown, provide assistance with balance and mobility, interrupt a panic attack, and seek help for an incapacitated handler, among other tasks. For some, this partnership can help the disabled individual negotiate the transition between fear and confidence, suspicion and trust, and, ultimately, illness and health.

In addition to the specific tasks that PSDs perform, the bond between the handler and the dog can be the window into recovery. As many dog lovers can attest, the presence of their dogs helps them feel calmer, more relaxed, and more open to venture out into the world and interact with others. Handlers report that their service dogs "center" them and make them "feel safe"; many no longer experience the overwhelming emptiness of being alone or feeling "disconnected" and out of place when they are working with their dogs. Just walking with the dog can help alleviate symptoms of depression. The Depression and Bipolar Support Alliance (DBSA) "strongly believes that Psychiatric Service Dogs have afforded many mentally disabled individuals to reach a new level of wellness and the opportunity to lead happy and productive lives." Maintaining a routine can help the handler to manage daily tasks and activities, and caring for the dog often leads to feelings of greater confidence, self-reliance, cooperation, and self-esteem.

These effects are more than simply emotional, however, and the physical benefits of the human-animal bond have been well documented. Numerous studies have revealed that contact with animals can lower blood pressure, pulse, and respiration rates, and reduce the perception of pain and discomfort. Wounds heal faster and recovery times are shortened. Living with animals increases survival rates for individuals with serious chronic conditions. (For more information about this research, see Resources pages 240-241.)

Initially, the concept of a psychiatric service dog was resisted by more traditional service dog organizations, so early advocates of

PSDs created their own advocacy groups to exchange information and began to assist others in training their own psychiatric
service dogs to meet their specific needs. Around the country,
dog trainers, mental health professionals, and clients began to
share information through publications, Websites, Internet
lists, bulletin boards, forums, and presentations at professional
conferences. Recently some organizations that had been training dogs for other disabilities have also begun to train dogs for
those with psychiatric disabilities addressing a need that has
grown with increasing numbers of returning combat veterans
experiencing severe symptoms of PTSD.

Today, PSDs are trained to perform a wide variety of tasks
for their handlers that generally fall into the categories of assisting in a medical crisis, providing assistance with the individual's
ongoing medical treatment, assisting the individual to cope with
emotional pressures in public, and providing a sense of safety
and security to the individual at home. They may routinely bring
food or medications to their handlers, be trained to dial 911 on a
special phone, assist their handlers in steadying themselves when
they are dizzy or have fallen, provide tactile stimulation, lead
their handlers away from crowds, strangers, and other dangers,
and summon help in an emergency. (A detailed list of the many
services PSDs perform can be found in Appendix 6.)

In the following chapters, we'll talk about how these dogs
are trained to complete these complex tasks and routines, but
one of the first questions I am often asked is: "What kind of
dog makes the best PSD?" There is no single right answer.
They can be large or small, calm or energetic, and any breed
or mix of breeds. Many different types of dogs, both purebreds

and shelter dogs, have successfully been trained for this service and were chosen on the basis of their potential to perform their jobs in an appropriate manner based on the disabled individual's lifestyle and his or her personal appeal. As we will see, the search can lead in many directions and take many wagging forms.

The Dog Makes the Difference

Celia and Scout

Celia, a young woman in her late 20s, had lived with depression her whole life, managing her daily affairs by "gritting my teeth and willing myself to go forward." After several years, however, Celia found herself sliding further into a deep depression, and she developed a tremor that shook her entire body. She couldn't gather what little energy she had, began to lose interest in eating, and struggled to go to work. Finally, although she had unsuccessfully tried therapy in the past, after weeks of cajoling from her boyfriend, in desperation she made an appointment with a therapist.

Celia held out little hope for the treatment until she discovered that her new therapist regularly brought her dog to the sessions as part of her practice. The dog would sit next to Celia, who would just sit quietly and pet her. At first, there was no eye contact with either the dog or therapist, and often Celia wouldn't speak at all. Now, Celia found herself opening up in her sessions and divulging the pain and anxiety she often felt but had never revealed to anyone else before. The therapist's dog seemed to give Celia the courage to speak, to discuss the painful details of her life. Often, Celia would simply focus on the dog and at times would almost forget the therapist was even present as she shared her feelings. Based on her history, Celia and her therapist agreed to start Celia on medication, but the drugs failed to alleviate her symptoms and the side effects were limiting. Seeing how Celia had opened up in her sessions, after several months Celia's therapist suggested that Celia consider working with a PSD of her own.

Celia had happy memories of the dogs she had had while growing up. On her 30th birthday she made a visit to her local ASPCA. Though the rows of cages elicited feelings of being trapped, helpless, and neglected, she was determined to find her dog. Although she had had male dogs in the past, Celia quickly honed in on a 4-year old female named Spike, a shepherd mix. Although the dog was underweight and cowering in the back of her cage, when Celia asked to meet Spike, the dog immediately ran to her, nuzzling her nose into Celia's belly. That was the beginning of her journey with the dog Celia renamed Scout.

Celia entered into the partnership with trepidation. She couldn't fathom how she could care for this living creature when she could barely care for herself, and, when Celia took the dog home, she found Scout to be a clingy and troublesome roommate. Despite their affectionate first greeting, Scout did not like to be touched, a trait Celia shared. Celia recognized the similarity in their temperaments right away. She also realized she did not have the slightest idea of how to care for the dog.

The saving grace for both of them were the long walks they shared. Before Scout entered Celia's life, she rarely went outside and now she was walking around in her neighborhood for hours a day. While they were out walking, people would often stop to chat with her about Scout, and Celia found herself interacting more frequently with other people. Celia and Scout attended obedience classes, which helped them learn to work as a team and soon they were known to everyone they met as "Scout and Celia." She then embarked on training Scout to perform tasks to assist her in coping better with anxiety attacks and other problems.

Scout always held her head high and seemed to know exactly where she was going and the most efficient way to get there without coming into contact with the bustling crowds around her. When Celia was experiencing severe anxiety levels and migraines, or when she was dissociating, Scout was trained with the cue "find home," a task that was reinforced through daily practice as they went to and from work. Celia frequently dropped things when she was experiencing tremors and she trained Scout to pick these items up for her to prevent her from getting dizzy or nauseous, and possibly falling. After a period of time, with reinforcement, Scout would automatically pick up dropped items from the floor and deliver them to Celia.

Perhaps the most valuable task Scout performed, one that helped alleviate Celia's agoraphobia and fear of being in public places, was to keep people at a distance in a crowded situation by blocking them from coming too close and invading Celia's space when she experienced high levels of anxiety. For example, Celia would ask Scout to watch her back, either by standing behind her or, for longer periods of time, lying down behind her in a position that prevented people from being able to approach Celia any closer from the rear than about three feet.

Celia also struggled with lack of motivation to eat when experiencing deep depression. Scout was trained to lead her to the refrigerator whenever she got up and to do a Sit-Stay in front of it until she opened the door. If she hadn't eaten for long stretches of time, seeing Scout patiently waiting there served as a vivid reminder she needed to eat and to positively reinforce this task. Scout also accompanied Celia when she ate meals in public. Once settled under a table in a restaurant, Scout became almost invisible. People were always startled when this dog would come popping out from underneath, exclaiming they didn't even know she was there. Celia no longer hid behind her cloak of invisibility as she and Scout made their way in the world.

Then Celia took the next step. Despite her disabilities, Celia had always managed to keep a job, but, when her disabilities began to interfere with her functioning at work, Celia made the difficult decision to have Scout accompany her to the office. Celia readily admitted that she was anxious about the questions that would arise over Scout's presence. With education, however, she found her coworkers receptive to Scout and understanding of her disabilities.

Scout was trained to lead Celia away from situations that were triggers, when Celia began to shake and have the tremors that were precursors to her panic attacks. The shakes and tremors Celia experienced out of increased anxiety were the cues Scout was trained to respond to. Scout would lead her out of that environment, a behavior that was reinforced, as this disrupted her symptoms and could sometimes prevent an on-coming panic attack. At work, when Celia's boss approached her and she was triggered, she would tell her boss that Scout needed to go outside to potty. Once Scout led her outside, if the tremors worsened instead of subsiding, Scout was taught to respond by leaning against her and nudging and pawing Celia to interrupt these tremors and convulsions. Scout would continue this task during the panic attack until Celia was no longer shaking and able to breathe normally again. This would prevent her from disassociating, and she'd be able to come back inside and return to work and focus.

In addition, Celia became an advocate for people with PSDs, including her rights as a disabled person to have Scout travel with her on the New York City subway. Since then, Celia and Scout have traveled all over the country, their world made ever larger as they face new experiences together. With Scout at her side Celia now faces conflicts head on with stoicism and pride.

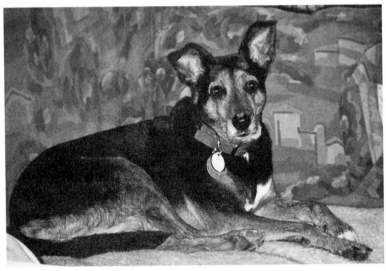

Scout, in repose after a day's work and long walk with Celia, remains attentive and ready for their next adventure.

Michele and Mordecai

Mordecai entered Michele's life one summer day as a stray, dreadlocked, flea-infested, 25-pound mystery mutt. At that time, Michele was a full-time college student sharing a house with four other girls. She had also just ended a very abusive relationship and had started dating a nice new man. After two weeks searching fruitlessly for the homeless dog's owner, Michele was thrilled to have this new-found companion. Michele named the little dog Mordecai and took him to a veterinarian, changed his diet, and walked him daily to teach him leash manners. Though he was people-shy, Michele and Mordecai bonded very quickly, and Michele spent endless hours training her new friend, never dreaming of the path he would lead her down in the months and years ahead.

With the help of a few friends, Mordecai became a very social dog and seemed to love people, and Michele decided to train Mordecai to be a therapy dog. Michele had planned to take Mordecai to hospitals and nursing homes to visit with the sick and elderly patients and residents. Michele attended classes given by the local Delta Society and used their reference books to train Mordecai for therapy dog work, and she brought Mordecai to pet-friendly stores to get him used to the stimuli of the world outside the home. Mordecai took it all in stride and enjoyed being out with Michele. He held his head high and wagged his tail. When Mordecai passed his therapy dog test, he was ready to work.

But while Michele and Mordecai's bond grew, Michele's relationship with her fiancé, Robin, was getting rocky, and one night, during a fight with her fiancé, Michele had a catharsis about her past. She realized she had been serially raped by a previous intimate partner and had buried memories of the abuse for three years. The trauma had been ruining her relationship with Robin. While she and Robin worked with a couple's therapist, Michele spent time in bed and suffered from a suffocating depression and an immobilizing fear of leaving her home. One day, Michele finally dragged herself out of bed and went with a friend to buy Mordecai some dog food at the pet store, where Michele's memories were triggered by a man who shared some of the same physical traits as her previous abusive partner. Michele found herself sitting on the floor of the pet store, curled into a ball.

Once Michele returned home, she took to the bed again. Michele hated not remembering what had happened, but her friend told Michele that she had some sort of "freak out" and that Mordecai had pawed at her over and over until it had stopped. Well, that accounted for the bad scratch on her leg, but how had Mordecai sensed her distress? While recuperating in bed, Michele did some research on PTSD and the work of service dogs for people with disabilities. She learned that some service dogs were trained to mitigate the effects of the handler's symptoms during a disassociative state. It was clear to Michele and her therapist that her PTSD, panic attacks, and depression were disabling, and she began to wonder if Mordecai could also be trained to mitigate the effects of her disability. She fit the ADA criteria as disabled and realized how the tasks Mordecai was being trained to perform diminished the effects of her symptoms.

As Michele sought help at her local Rape Crisis Center, Mordecai attended the therapy sessions with her. In the first stage of her healing, Michele was constantly triggered, experiencing frequent flashbacks, nightmares, hypervigilance, crippling anxiety, and constant emotional flux. Like Celia, when Michele suffered an attack, she would start shaking from head to toe. Mordecai immediately responded by pawing her until Michele was able to breath normally again and begin to function. Michele reinforced Mordecai's response to these cues and trained him to shape his alerts with gentler pawing so he did not scratch her. He also was trained to use his nose to alert her when she was collapsed on the floor by placing his nose on her chin and nudging it until she would look up, continuing to nudge until Michele was capable of standing up without losing her balance. When Michele returned to school, Mordecai's assistance was invaluable. His alerts helped her to focus on her schoolwork and not on the stresses wreaking havoc on her emotions.

Mordecai was soon helping Michele in other ways as well. Michele rode the bus to and from school every day and Michele trained him to sit under her seat on his mat. The bus was often crowded, and Michele found the crowds raised her anxiety level. In an attempt to cope, Michele wore headphones and sunglasses to block out her surroundings, which occasionally caused her to miss her stop. Once Mordecai had a pattern set of which stops they used and was cued to find home, he learned to alert Michele when their stop was coming up by standing up and pawing her. With Michele's praise, Mordecai began to alert for their stop more reliably.

With Mordecai's assistance, Michele has graduated from college with a double degree in music and religious studies and now has a fulfilling full-time job. Mordecai accompanies Michele to the office, where this little dog fits snugly in his bed under her desk, and Michele's coworkers are welcoming to Mordecai and accepting of Michele's disability. The small, plucky dog has adjusted to living with Robin and Michele and their other pets in their small apartment, and is happy to cuddle with Michele when she just wants to lay around the house. On the day she found him, Michele could not have imagined that this scruffy, homeless mutt would not only assist her in getting out of her bed to face the world, but that with Mordecai's help she would be able to graduate from college, hold down a job, enjoy a healthy relationship with her husband, and cope with the ups and downs of daily life. In Michele's words, "Mordecai has prevented me from letting my panic disorder and PTSD stop me from having a rich and fulfilling life!"

Although PSDs must learn the basic service skills that other service dogs share, they must also be sensitive to the thoughts and feelings of their partners, and be trained for specific tasks that mitigate the effects of that individual's disability. Although their dogs performed different tasks, Celia and Michele benefited from dogs that displayed calm, reassuring temperaments. For other individuals, like Micky and Nancy, a more energetic dog proved to be just what they needed.

Micky and Jake

Micky fled her family at age 19 after suffering from years of physical, emotional, and sexual abuse. By age 22, she was "your basic depressed and defensive childhood incest survivor," as she puts it. The pattern of mistreatment continued well into her 30s, with boyfriends and lovers who were physically abusive and emotionally manipulative. It was Jake, a bullmastiff puppy, that changed her life; he became her anchor, her protector, her teacher, her confidant, and, ultimately, in her words, "my guardian angel." Bullmastiffs are enormous dogs, difficult to navigate in public places, and not the first type that comes to mind for the ideal service dog. However, once again, the unlikely proved to be the best option.

Micky was living in a loft in Brooklyn, working part-time as a dog trainer, when her boyfriend suggested she get an eye-catching dog to help promote her business. After meeting a lost bullmastiff at the local shelter, Micky knew this was the type of dog for her. She contacted a breeder in Virginia who had a new littler of pups, and when she met him, puppy Jake passed his aptitude tests with flying colors. Proving himself to be resilient, confident, and compliant, Jake would be the perfect personal companion and dog training assistant. But, more importantly, it seemed to Micky that Jake had the potential to fit into Micky's plan of volunteering with her dog to visit institutionalized individuals. So four days later, Jake went home to Brooklyn with Micky.

Within days of his arrival, however, Jake became extremely ill with distemper and parvo virus, contracted from his vaccinations. Micky braced herself for the worst, as puppies younger than 12 weeks rarely survived these diseases. But the feisty Jake survived. Jake continued to experience additional health problems, but Micky rose to the occasion everytime and the crises just seemed to strengthen her bond with the dog. She marveled at his resilience and determination, stating that he had "all the things I was lacking."

Micky began training Jake, and, as he became more proficient, he was entered in dog shows and obedience trials so he could work on his service dog skills and be exposed to high pressure situations. Micky even showed Jake at the prestigious Westminster Kennel Club show at Madison Square Garden in New York. Whatever Micky thought up, Jake could do. He went to work with her, helped her in her dog training classes, and still had energy to spare for field trips and outings to the grocery store, mall, and all of the other places Micky could have never gone to alone.

As she began to work with Jake, Micky recognized that, to be a truly competent care-giver, she needed to be physically and mentally healthy herself. Jake's early illnesses made it clear to Micky, who had struggled with anorexia, that serious nutrition was essential, not only for Jake, but for herself as well. Feeding Jake reminded her to eat regularly and helped her to think of food as a source of nourishment.

During the course of Jake's training, Micky noted that many of her physical ailments diminished or abated. Her motto became "dog + woman = less stress," which translated into fewer migraines, return of appetite, less back pain, and no more asthma. Now when she had a migraine, rather than taking to her bed, she went though her day, business as usual, relying on Jake for assistance. If the migraine became blinding, Jake would help her navigate the crowded streets of New York City by following directional commands such as "Forward, Left, Right, Serpentine, and Halt."

Whenever Micky felt a panic attack coming on, Jake was trained to rest his big head in her lap on the command "Lay Keppie," and she'd match her breaths to his as she stroked his chest. This process leveled out Micky's emotions so that she could regain her composure. In addition, this strategy sometimes abated the symptoms of an oncoming migraine.

Jake was also trained to provide counter-balance support for Micky when her anxiety levels and panic caused her instability. He made it possible for her to ambulate without falling due to her fears and the increased level of stress she experienced. If the severity of the panic attack made it too risky for her to walk, Jake could help Micky to reach the nearest bench or place to sit down.

Jake's size, energy, and demeanor met Micky's needs. She was now able to work at a full-time job, participate in a volunteer program, and take an assortment of classes. Because of her dog, Micky overcame her years of social anxiety and hypervigilance. She started behavioral therapy and began attending Al-Anon meetings. Simple daily activities, such as taking a walk or going on a hike, no longer filled her with anxiety because her competent and confident dog was at her side.

Nancy and Windy

Nancy also discovered that an exuberant, curious, energetic dog was the right match and partner for her. Nancy had purchased Windy, a "Nova Scotia Duck Tolling Retriever" puppy from a breeder simply to be a companion, but when Windy was about three years old, she startled Nancy one day by leaping into her lap while Nancy was having a panic attack, wrapping her front legs around Nancy's shoulders and resting on her chest until Nancy's symptoms began to subside. After some experimentation with this novel interaction, Nancy decided to train Windy to perform this highly desirable behavior on command. She discovered that the weight of Windy on her torso and abdomen, while she lay on the couch or floor, as well as the distracting softness of Windy's fur as Windy lay her head against Nancy's, not only prevented her symptoms from escalating, but also seemed to shorten the duration of the panic attack. The dog's weight provided what later would become known as "deep pressure therapy," which has been shown to have a calming effect on children and adults with autism and other individuals who suffer from severe panic attacks.

Nancy's prior experience as a trainer also enabled her to train Windy to keep Nancy at a safe distance from other people in crowded situations in public. Windy was able to sense fluctuations in Nancy's stress levels, and Nancy channeled the dog's reaction into a practical task. Nancy taught Windy, whenever she sensed that Nancy was starting to feel panicky and dissociating, to lead Nancy to her parked car when she was unable to locate it herself. After many months of practice, Windy now is able to find the car in crowded parking lots with ease.

Nancy learned that Windy's natural ability to detect the onset of her panic episodes could be enhanced and reinforced through scent discrimination training. Windy was soon able to alert Nancy to an impending attack, and Nancy has consistently reinforced this useful behavior. Windy was not able to stop the attacks, but the interruptive quality of the tasks that she is trained to perform at such times has been a huge relief and great mitigating force. Prior to Windy entering Nancy's life, she would feel exhausted and immobilized for hours after these debilitating episodes. The assistance of her service dog has significantly shortened her recovery time.

Nonetheless, Nancy realized that she needed to find a way to relieve Windy's energetic nature, and they both fell in love with a variety of dog sports. Though these activities were intended for Windy's benefit, they also forced Nancy out into the world, where she interacted with other dog handlers and trainers. Windy, in turn, now had an outlet for her excessive

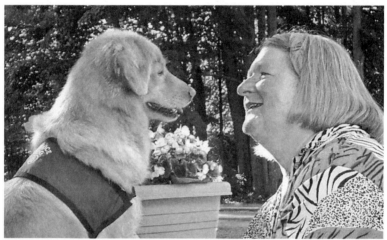

Watchful Windy, so intuitive, is ever on the alert to Nancy's feelings and needs, and Nancy tries to reciprocate with her admiration, attention, and affection.

energy. Although others might find Windy's temperament high strung, her strong reaction to stimuli enable her to detect Nancy's physical/emotional symptoms and help lessen her attacks, and when Nancy needs her, she is calm and up for the task.

Tracy, Finola, and Baron

Feeling unhappy in her long-term relationship, Tracy believed that she and her partner would benefit if they explored their problems together. After their first session, however, she recognized that she wanted to pursue therapy on her own. This was a huge step for Tracy, who had relied on her partner for nearly everything, but after a number of months Tracy realized that her partner controlled every aspect of her life. Tracy had never grocery shopped or entered a bank by herself. At the beginning of their lives together, this arrangement had worked, but Tracy now admitted to herself how imbalanced and abusive her relationship was, and broke up with her partner. Expecting to be happier with her new-found independence, instead Tracy now discovered her own helplessness. She was terrified of going out into the world, but felt trapped within the confines of her home, struggling to eat, sleep, cook, clean, and function without experiencing debilitating panic and fear. Simply getting through her days was an ordeal.

During our therapy sessions, Tracy, like Mindy, was inspired by Umaya's strength, courage, and unconditional love, sensing how attuned Umaya was to her every fluctuation in mood. Tracy decided that she, too, would like to adopt a psychiatric service dog and wanted a labrador retriever because they are so commonly seen as guide dogs and thus less likely to elicit public curiosity and questions. Tracy already owned two dogs, a Pomeranian and a Boxer, but these dogs were elderly and frail, not appropriate candidates for the service she required. She knew she could not train or cope with a high-strung puppy and wanted to find a Labrador that was at least 2 years old, a dog that would have a little less energy but was young enough to go through the training process and work for many years as her PSD.

Tracy learned about Baron when an advertisement in the local newspaper listed a retired stud dog that needed a home. As she drove to meet him, Tracy was filled with hopeful anticipation and anxiety but was heartbroken at his condition when she found him living in a filthy overcrowded barn. Baron was infested with fleas, wounded by bug bites, and suffering from a torn and infected ear. Tracy knew immediately, however, that she had to save him. She recognized the risks of adopting a dog from these harsh conditions, but identified with his situation, having been adopted as an infant from a tumultuous situation herself.

After taking Baron home, Tracy knew that the first step was to address his physical needs. Tracy went directly to a veterinarian who repaired Baron's ear, and he began a regimen of antibiotics and other medications. Baron healed rapidly and he began to trust Tracy, who, in turn, felt capable of taking care of another being although she was struggling to take care of herself.

Within a brief time, Baron had adjusted to his new home and it became apparent he already had quite a bit of training under his belt. Baron knew basic behaviors—sit, come, stay, and even heel to some degree. Tracy started the process of training Baron, taking him for classes in basic obedience and a Canine Good Citizen class. Baron was a pro at the obedience training and had a calm, gentle temperament that seemed to draw Tracy out. When in public, Tracy was able to have brief interactions with the people who stopped to admire Baron and comment on how well-behaved he was. Tracy felt liberated because the focus wasn't on her but on her dog, and her confidence and self-esteem were bolstered. Soon, Tracy and I were taking him out to local restaurants, movie theaters, elevators, banks, grocery stores, and so on. And specifically training him to mitigate the effects of Tracy's disability. Tracy and Baron were off to a good start.

It soon became clear, however, that Baron intuitively picked up on Tracy's deep depression and anxiety. Baron's mood

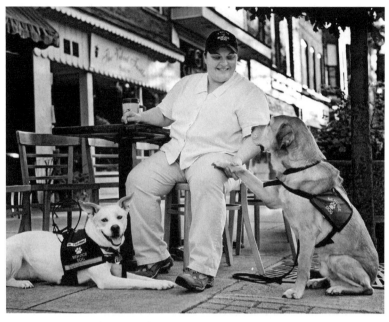

Tracy, out for an afternoon meal while training. Baron, her PSD, is demonstrating for Finola, her PSDIT how to paw her when having difficulty coping with the crowds of people strolling through town.

began to mirror Tracy's lethargy and lack of motivation, and he seemed to want to leave a new situation immediately after entering. Now anticipating the dog's discomfort, Tracy's anxiety level increased even more than usual, and their mutual fear of public places was only exacerbating the problem. After Baron had spent several months as Tracy's Psychiatric Service Dog in Training, we both recognized that, in Tracy's words, "Baron isn't enjoying his job." The training had reached a standstill; neither Tracy nor Baron were making progress.

After weeks of deliberation, Tracy and I concluded that the best option was to give Baron a break from his PSD duties. We both knew that it takes very particular skills to diminish the effects of a disability, and not every dog is meant for the job. This is a reality of adopting, training, and finding the right service dog. There are no certainties, but, as Tracy discovered, Baron was nonetheless a part of her recovery process. He had helped her begin to face the world—no small feat.

Tracy was now ready for her next Psychiatric Service Dog and was starting to feel less depressed, more energetic, and committed to the training process. Realizing that she and Baron fed off each other's complacent, slow, sad demeanors, Tracy knew she needed a dog with a radically different temperament. Fast-forward to her next PSD, a boisterous, fun-loving, entertaining white mutt named Finola (Gaelic for "white shoulder"). Finola was one of the many uprooted survivors of Hurricane Katrina who now needed a permanent home.

Tracy wanted a dog that would help motivate her to take longer walks and be more energetic, and she immediately recognized that Finola was full of exuberance. In a short time, however, Finola began to calm down as Tracy and I took weekly walks with Finola, parallel walking with my two Golden Retrievers to help Finola adapt to being around other dogs and learn to heel by mirroring their actions. Tracy learned how to communicate with Finola, how to be consistent, and how to reinforce appropriate behaviors. It was a slow, deliberate process that required enormous patience as Finola was trained to mitigate the effects of Tracy's disability by nudging her when she was disassociating, pulling her out of an uncomfortable situation, placing her paws on Tracy's feet to help her focus, or standing behind her to provide a buffer to prevent strangers from standing too close. All of these techniques provided security as Tracy faced her fears out in public places.

Finola was also trained to disrupt Tracy's obsessive/compulsive behaviors when she spent too much time at the computer or too many hours watching television. In these cases, Finola would lead Tracy away from whatever activity Tracy had been doing for hours to break up her compulsive pattern. Finola was trained to pick up on Tracy's increasing anxiety level and was then reinforced for interrupting these symptoms. When Tracy was feeling emotional, she would turn to food for comfort, and Finola was trained to prevent Tracy from overeating by nudging and pawing her to get her up to leave the food and take her for a walk. This task was reinforced by the trainer and Tracy for a number of months, until Finola immediately responded to Tracy's elevated stress level while either eating compulsively or obsessively sitting in front of the computer or television.

For Tracy the entire training process was therapeutic. Initially, Tracy did not bond with either of her dogs quickly due to her history of abuse. She was wary of trusting anyone, even a dog. Over time, we worked on her patting her dogs, giving them massages, and, after months of living together, even cuddling with them. Tracy was slowly and cautiously learning how to care for another being with love, something that had terrified her in the past. As Tracy nurtured Finola and Baron, the bonds of trust and affection grew stronger.

Every handler has different needs that are subject to change over time, and it is critical to continue to reassess those needs to find the right match. When it works, a PSD is a wondrous prescription for a fulfilling life. Baron had helped Tracy gain confidence and started her on her journey outward into the world again. Baron's respite from service was healing and he is now thoroughly enjoying returning to brief episodes of work on Finola's days off. Finola's energy and adventurous nature help Tracy to take risks previously unimaginable as they navigate new territory together. Today Tracy and Finola educate others about PSDs, lecturing to audiences of more than 100 medical professionals, a possibility no one could have imagined just a few years ago.

Which Dog Is Right for You?

Different breeds, different temperaments, different tasks, different dogs. No one dog is right for every circumstance or even every individual at different points in his or her life. Though traditional service dogs are often drawn from a handful of breeds, experience has shown that dogs of many stripes can make wonderful PSDs. They can be purebred or shelter dogs; obtained from breeders or foster homes; raised and trained from puppyhood or adopted as older dogs with some life experience and training already under their belts. Male or female, large or small, with some sensitive screening and careful planning, many ordinary dogs can make an extraordinary difference in the lives of someone with emotional disabilities. The most important qualities are the health, temperament, and intelligence of the potential PSD candidate.

Before seeking out you potential PSD, I suggest that you write out a "job description" that details your environment and circumstances and outlines the service requirements for your potential candidate. This description would take into account your:

- Lifestyle: whether you are single, partnered, married, have children, or live with other extended family members.
- Pets: whether you have other dogs, cats, birds, pocket pets, and small mammals (rabbits, guinea pigs, etc.)
- Type of housing: whether you live in an apartment, townhouse, single family house, or other type of dwelling.
- Location: Whether you live in a rural, urban, or suburban area.
- Job: what are the requirements of your occupation or profession.
- Hobbies: the other activities you and your family engage in regularly.
- Frequency of travel: how often you need to travel by car, bus, subway, or air.
- Level of activity: sedentary versus high energy level.
- Dog "smarts": whether you are a novice or experienced dog owner, or if you have successfully trained or maintained the training of a dog.

Additionally, you need to itemize the tasks the dog will perform to mitigate the effects of your disability. As with any "job search," the candidate that most closely matches the requirements established in your job description is the best dog for the job.

Meeting and observing your prospective PSD is essential! I highly recommend that if you are not adopting your dog from a program that specifically trains PSDs that you find a trainer who has previous experience in training service dogs to help you select your dog, whether from a breeder, a foster home, a shelter, or choosing a retired show dog (who is not too old) or a service dog who didn't complete training as a guide dog or hearing dog for reasons other than health issues but might make a good PSD. This individual can go over your "job description" with you and assist you in finding the right dog to suit your needs. The trainer should have experience in temperament testing, and can look specifically for signs of aggressiveness, shyness, friendliness, how the dog reacts to strangers, noises, visual stimuli, different floor substrates, and many other situations that can help indicate whether or not the dog has the potential to be a PSD. Unless you are willing to take on challenges of raising a puppy, you will probably be looking at a dog between 2 and 3 years of age. At this age, the dog can be tested for hereditary diseases characteristic of its breed, while allowing for training time and a partnership that will last for years to come.

Once you have narrowed down your choices, I suggest that you request an overnight stay with your potential service dog. Try to play games with the dog, like hiding treats to assess the dog's level of curiosity, persistence, and ability to figure things out, and observe how the dog adapts and copes with the new environment. The service dog needs to be confident, resilient, compliant, focused, not easily distracted, and able to focus on you even if there are other people present. Service dogs are not rehabilitation projects, so starting out with a dog who is not sound sensitive, fearful, or reactive is a must. Above all, your PSD should be selected for its ability to assist you.

Here are some things to consider when choosing your PSD:

1. What kind of dogs do you like? This is a very good place to start. If you've had a dog before, you may already know that you like small plucky dogs or big shaggy ones, that you love fuzzy coats or black noses, or prefer beagles, or boxers, or labs. Bonding to the dog is a must—this is a partnership filled with love and respect—and you may already be open to certain breeds and looks. Keep in mind, however, that your service dog will be more than a pet; he or she will be a professional, with a serious job to perform. Be aware that your circumstances may have changed, the type of dog you're looking for may not be available or be best suited to your needs, and that many other wonderful dogs with just the right qualities may now be better equipped for the job. I highly recommend reading Joan Froling's *Finding a Suitable Candidate for Assistance Dog Work*, which can be found at *www.iaadp. org/breed.html* for breed choice information. (For even more information, see Appendix 4 and the Resources pages 236-237.)

2. Is size a consideration? This may be a matter of preference, convenience, and control. If you want your dog to assist you in navigating through crowds and strange environments, a larger dog might be a good option. Or you may feel that a larger dog would be difficult to handle and a smaller dog is more manageable. Can your home or office accommodate a large dog without feeling cramped? If you need to travel often, will your dog fit comfortably on planes, trains, buses, and

so on? Remember that your dog will be working with you in public. A large dog with a long tail will have to be trained to tuck it under in stores to avoid knocking items off of shelves or to prevent being stepped upon. Consider the tasks you will need the dog to perform to mitigate the effects of your disability, which may help you clarify the size of the dog you require. Remember that the lifespan of most larger dogs is shorter than for smaller dogs.

3. Are grooming and bathing issues for you? If so, you should look at dogs that need minimal grooming and don't have long coats that might easily mat. Dogs with heavy coats may also require additional grooming during the hot summer. In addition to the time, effort, and expense you may expend on dog-grooming, your dog is going out into public places and should always be clean and look his or her best.

4. Which dog has the best temperament for you? As we've seen, some people require an energetic dog to urge them to remain active and outgoing, whereas others prefer the calming influence of a more serene temperament. Although dogs are individuals, there are strong breed tendencies in temperament. Research breeds at the American Kennel Club (*www.akc.org/breeds* and see Appendix 4 and Resources pages 236-237) so you have some idea of what the dog's most common traits might be and if they will best fit your needs. Behavioral characteristic such as hunting instincts and barking can be problematic. Do you need a dog that's gentle with

children? Would an aggressive dog get along with your other pets? Are some breed types known to be "quick learners"? Outgoing and friendly? very protective of their handlers? Extremely loyal?

Large terriers, working, or guarding breed-types are often seen as aggressive by shopkeepers, security personnel, and others, which can cause unnecessary confrontation, whereas hounds and toy dogs are thought by some to be unfocused and "not smart enough" to work as service dogs. Even if the dog you're considering is a wonderful mutt, it is still helpful to have an idea of its makeup (hound mix, bull/terrier mix, herding/retriever mix) to know which traits the dog might exhibit. Also remember that the dog's history affects its personality. Emotionally, a well-cared-for dog that was responsibly surrendered to a shelter or a rescue group may be more appropriate than a rescue dog that was picked up as a stray. Solid temperament— that is, a resilient and confident dog—supersedes everything else.

5. Do you want a puppy or an older dog? Can you handle the energy and training that owning a new puppy entails? Can you wait for the dog to reach emotional maturity, which for most dogs is 18 to 24 months of age? If you're getting a puppy, the dog may show stronger breed tendencies out of the gate than if you're adopting an older dog that may have experienced some knocks in life before meeting you. An older dog may be calmer, but may also come with some baggage and bad habits,

as well as be beginning to demonstrate health concerns, such as problems with the hips and joints. You want to consider the age of the dog as well as the time the training will take to ensure that you and the dog have a lengthy partnership.

6. Are there additional costs related to the kind of dog you want? Once you've committed to the cost of supporting a healthy PSD, you will be responsible for veterinary care, equipment and training costs, food, grooming, play toys, and other miscellaneous items. Expenditures may vary depending on the size, breed, age, temperament, and so on, of the dog. Although some organizations are able to help defray some of these costs, every dog handler will have out-of-pocket expenses.

Give yourself time to observe your dog's behavior before making a decision. If possible, spend as much time as you can with the dog outside of the cage to see how it responds to gestures and commands. Does it like to be touched? Is it easily distracted? Can it focus? Dogs that are anxious, sensitive, fearful, or easily startled are not appropriate candidates for the life of a service dog, which can be demanding and stressful. Make sure you take someone with you who has experience training dogs, is familiar with temperament testing, and specifically knows your psychiatric needs to help evaluate your dog's potential. It takes a special dog to fulfill the challenging job of a PSD, but finding "your dog" can be a life-changing event.

3

The Good Fight: Prison Puppies Free Veterans From Combat

Throughout our nation's history, we have experienced the tragedy of veterans returning from war with physical wounds and facing lifelong disabilities. Fortunately, many government and private organizations exist to help these men and women return to civilian life. In this effort, service dogs have long been paired with physically disabled veterans to assist them in their daily lives. In more recent years, however, psychiatric service dogs have helped many veterans deal with the scars of war that are far more difficult to see.

The condition of Post-Traumatic Stress Disorder (PTSD) first became well known after an alarming number of veterans returned from the Vietnam War in the 1960s and 1970s with disturbing symptoms of emotional stress. Now recognized as a specific condition, PTSD is characterized, according to the

DSM-IV guidelines, by "recurrent and intrusive distressing recollections of the event, including images, thoughts or perceptions, recurrent distressing dreams of the event, [or] acting or feeling as if the traumatic event were recurring." These experiences might include "a sense of reliving the experience, illusions, hallucinations and dissociative flashback episodes including those that occur on awakening or when intoxicated, intense psychological distress at exposure to internal or external cues that symbolize or resemble an aspect of the traumatic event." In addition, the individual may have trouble sleeping, be irritable or prone to anger, have difficulty concentrating, and be easily startled. It's as if the person suffering from PTSD is always expecting the traumas associated with the past to reoccur and is therefore often anxious and wary.

More recently, veterans of the Gulf Wars and the wars in Iraq and Afghanistan have also displayed the symptoms of PTSD. In this chapter, two veterans will share their stories about their experiences today with psychiatric service dogs that they obtained through two different service dog training programs. Like many other individuals, these men found these animals to have virtually saved their lives.

In 2006, Raymond Hubbard's unit of the Wisconsin National Guard was called up for action in Iraq. When Raymond left for Iraq, his wife, Sarah, wanted him to focus on everything that would be waiting for him upon his return and promised that when he came back he could get a dog, like he'd had when he was a boy. As he left for his tour, Raymond never dreamed that six months later he would return home after surviving a horrific injury.

Conditions in Iraq were difficult and dangerous. Just months after he arrived, under intense fire during a July 4th raid in Baghdad, Raymond was hammered with shrapnel that amputated his left leg below his knee and damaged his ability to use his right arm. His carotid artery was severed causing a massive stroke, and he spent three weeks in a coma. Both the stroke and the coma had caused permanent damage to his brain. In addition, he was unable to speak due to the effects of the stroke and damage to his vocal cords.

Raymond had grown up in a family of veterans. There was no question in his mind that he would continue this tradition of serving his country. His father, brother, uncle, and two grandfathers had served in the military, and Raymond didn't hesitate to join the ranks. In fact, his father had been severely wounded 40 years earlier in Vietnam and had never fully recovered emotionally or physically from his wounds. He died when Raymond was 14 from alcoholism and suspected complications from exposure to Agent Orange. He had been an abusive alcoholic, and the home felt unsafe and terrifying for Raymond, who survived his turbulent teenage years with his beloved dog, Chunker, by his side. "Chunker saved my life on more than one occasion when I felt suicidal," Hubbard recalls, "by placing a lick on my face or begging for some play time. Now that I'm 30, I look back and realize I was mostly not myself when I was a man without a dog."

After emergency surgery at Landstuhl Hospital in Germany, Raymond was transferred to the Walter Read Army Medical Center in Bethesda, Maryland. Overwhelmed by his losses, Raymond had trouble organizing his life, concentrating, and speaking, and he descended into depression. He was on enormous quantities of pain killers, spending his days sleeping and fending off terrifying nightmares. Raymond knew he did not want to end up like his father, and he wanted his children to grow up with a loving, gentle, healthy dad and husband. His injuries, however, made him feel helpless.

One day, while lying in his hospital bed at Walter Reed, a Golden Retriever in a therapy dog vest entered his room with his trainer. Although Raymond could barely speak, the connection that he felt with the dog was immediate and profound. When the occupational therapist saw Raymond's elated reaction, she suggested he contact the National Education of Assistance Dog Services (NEADS), a center that has helped hundreds of disabled individuals live more independently at home, work, and school to see if he would be eligible for one of their programs.

NEADS, located on an 18-acre campus in Princeton, Massachusetts, was established in 1976 to provide puppies and dogs to assist those who are deaf or physically disabled, and since its founding has trained more than 1,300 service dogs and rescue dogs. In addition to helping the disabled, the NEADS Prison PUP Partnership employs inmates in 14 correctional facilities throughout New England training canines for NEADS, plus more than 30 foster families training canines in their homes for the NEADS programs.

Sheila O'Brien, NEADS previous Chief Executive Officer, has found that this program benefits the prisoners, the dogs, and the veterans. The puppies, mostly Labradors and golden retrievers, spend about 18 months training at the prison, learning more than 70 commands before they are ready for their more specialized training. Nonetheless, the training the dogs receive from the inmates takes half the time it would in foster homes due to the unlimited time the inmates have to spend with the puppies. At the same time, the inmates appreciate being able to do useful work and gain a sense of self-worth through the program. In addition, the corrections officers have reported that the presence of these dogs has had a positive impact reducing stress and improving the overall prison environment.

In September 2006, Sheila started the Canines for Combat Veterans program, recognizing the increasing need of veterans with combat injuries. All costs for veterans are covered by NEADS, the dogs training, healthcare and all of the expenses covered by NEADS are approximately $20,000. Raymond was accepted into the NEADS program and given a black Labrador Retriever named Dace, who had been trained as a puppy by Barbara Goucher, a prisoner at the State Prison For Women in Framingham, Massachusetts. Dace was born at the Guiding Eyes for the Blind Canine Development Center, but because she was too feisty and sound-sensitive to be a guide dog, she was transferred at 16 weeks old to MCI-Framingham (Massachusetts Correctional Institute in Framingham) for the program. Dace was specifically trained to assist Raymond with his mobility disability, but, with the training Raymond received during his two weeks at NEADS, he also learned how to task train Dace to assist him with his PTSD symptoms.

As he started the program, Raymond was informed by the trainer that there was a chance that he and Dace wouldn't take to each other, and Raymond remembers that he had "never worried about someone liking me as much as with this life-changing canine." Raymond was extremely apprehensive the first time he met Dace and showered her with treats, but she seemed cautious and wary of leaving the trainer's side. Raymond's heart sank with the thought that they weren't going to bond, that the chemistry just wasn't right. It wasn't until the third day when Raymond was throwing a ball for Dace that she ran back to him instead of the trainer. "It was magical," Raymond recalled.

Dace soon displayed her ability to assist Raymond with his PTSD symptoms. One day, as he was visiting the National Air Space Museum in Washington, D.C., he and his sons were watching an Omnimax film about jet fighter planes. When a rocket blew up on the screen, Raymond had a flashback of being attacked in Iraq and couldn't breathe. He was gasping for air and about to pass out when Dace jumped up from his feet, nudging Raymond, licking his face and arms vigorously until he was able to breathe normally again and his tunnel vision evaporated. As some research has shown, PSDs have been shown to have a calming effect on their handlers, helping to stave off or lessen the effects of panic and anxiety. At that moment Raymond realized how much more Dace could be trained to do in addition to assisting him with his mobility.

Raymond still experiences episodes of paranoia and fear, but Dace has learned to help Raymond alleviate those feelings in numerous ways. Dace has been trained to search, upon entering the house, all of the rooms and return to let Raymond know all is safe. She has also been trained to find his bottles of pills when his severe symptoms of attention deficit disorder prevent him from remembering where he has placed them.

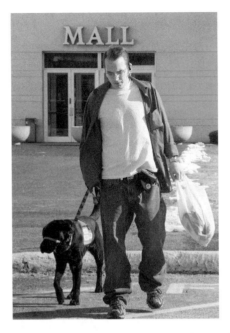

Iraq War veteran Raymond with Dace, his PSD, wearing her service vest. Dace's support and training help Raymond accomplish everyday tasks with greater confidence.

When Raymond is sleeping fitfully, Dace awakens him from his terrible dreams, nudging him to get out of bed and watch TV until his nightmares have passed. "If I didn't have Dace," Raymond says, "I would be isolated in my home. She gets me out into the world and leads me into the veterans' hospital rooms to empower other veterans by her presence. Dace was originally trained as my mobility service dog, but she wears so many more hats then that."

For Hubbard, Goucher, and Dace it has been a long journey. Goucher is especially proud of the work she has been able to do with NEADS. "My troubled life had come full circle when I met a soldier who will be helped by Dace," she says. "I have a better purpose. The dog contributed to that. It changed my life. It calmed me down. It was an honor to raise this dog for him." Dace has given Raymond independence and helped in the important work of his life by assisting him in his mission to educate other veterans about service dogs. Raymond's dream growing up was to be a public speaker and now he travels across the country with Dace, educating other veterans about the NEADS program and the gift Dace has been in his life. As his wife promised, when Raymond returned from combat he got his dog and so much more.

Back in 1980, at 18 years of age, Bill Campbell felt his only option to escape his abusive home life in the small suburb of Lacey, Washington, was to enlist in the Army. He spent 10 years in the Washington Army National Guard, first as a military photographer and then as a commissioned artillery officer. Bill was honorably discharged in 1990. While Bill was still serving in the Guard, he received his bachelor's degree in biology in 1986 from Evergreen State College. That same year he began his 19-year career with the Department of Fish and Wildlife as a Fish Biologist. In 2001, Bill went on to get his master's degree in public administration, also from the Evergreen State College. At the time he was happily married and living with his wife and three children.

When his former guard unit of 10 years was deployed to Iraq in 2004, Bill felt compelled to re-enlist. At age 45, he felt a sense of obligation to the institution that had provided him with healthcare, an education, and training that had bolstered his self-confidence and allowed him to pursue an interesting career. He also believed his experience and maturity would help him educate and possibly save other soldiers' lives.

Bill was stationed in Baghdad as a security guard at a base in the center of the city, where he was subject to daily crossfire, sniper attacks, car bombings, and firefights. In the midst of such a constant barrage, he was injured twice from shrapnel from car bombs, which injured his head and hand, producing traumatic brain injury (TBI) and severe nerve damage. The injuries that were the most debilitating, however, were the psychological ones, including severe anxiety, depression, jumpiness, intrusive memories, nightmares, paranoia, hallucinations, hyper-vigilance, memory problems, attention deficit disorder, and agoraphobia, all symptoms of PTSD.

When Bill returned from Iraq in 2005, he spent several weeks at a veterans hospital in Washington state before returning to the work he loved, but in less than six months it became apparent that he could barely function, let alone hold a job. He was sent to the PTSD inpatient unit at the Seattle Veterans Hospital for treatment. Bill underwent two and a half weeks of intensive treatment to address his PTSD symptoms. His relationship with his wife, who had trouble adjusting to the changes in his personality brought on by his disability, was extremely stressful, and they divorced within in a year of Bill's return home. When Bill started seeing a psychologist through the Veterans Administration, the therapist suggested that Bill consider a program called "Puppies Behind Bars (PBB)." The therapist thought a dog would relieve his isolation by getting him out of the house and helping him cope with his severe PTSD symptoms. Bill hadn't grown up with dogs and never was drawn to them, but he was willing now to try anything and he contacted the director of the PBB program.

PBB was established in 1997 by Gloria Gilbert Stoga after she adopted Arrow, a Labrador Retriever, from "Guiding Eyes For The Blind." Arrow had been released from the program due to physical ailments, but Gloria was impressed with what Arrow had learned and how well trained he was already. Gloria

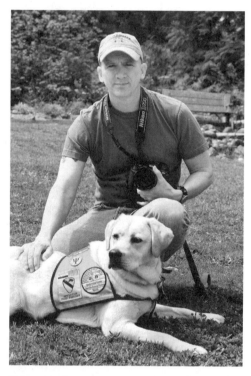

William Campbell and his service dog and best buddy, Pax, out for a day of photography.

was intrigued by the breeding and training process, and was deeply impressed by the amount of time, love, money, and effort that went into the training of every single guide dog. Gloria continued her research and learned that Dr. Thomas Lane, a veterinarian from Florida, had launched a program in which puppies were being raised by inmates for service as guide dogs.

Based on her experience with Arrow, Gloria was inspired to quit her job to start her own non-profit organization dedicated to training prisoners to raise puppies for the blind. Since the inception of the program with five puppies placed behind bars at the Bedford Hills Correctional Facility in New York, PBB has now expanded to seven correctional facilities raising more than 100 puppies at any one time. The organization has placed more than 550 puppies as service dogs for individuals with a diverse range of disabilities. After 9/11, Gloria introduced the Explosive Detection Canine Program because of the expanding need for canines to detect bombs and has now placed dogs with the NYPD Bomb Squad.

More recently, Gloria also started a program for the veterans returning home from Iraq and Afghanistan with PTSD, TBI, and physical injuries called "Dog Tags: Service Dogs for Those Who've Served Us." PBB provides service dogs to veterans free of charge. Like the NEADS program, the organization covers all of the costs ranging from raising and training the puppies to the expenses of the veterans' two-week team training program. Room, board, and transportation to the facility are all covered. In February 2008, Bill became the first candidate to adopt a PSD through PBB.

Although Bill never had an affinity for dogs, a yellow Labrador Retriever named Pax (Latin for "peace") has transformed his life. (Unlike many other individuals who have shared their stories in this book, Bill's experience illustrates that a previous connection to dogs is not necessary to discover the potential benefits of a PSD.) Before adopting Pax, Bill was reclusive, rarely went outside of his home, lived in constant fear, was overtaken by paranoia, terrified of strangers, and experienced nightly hallucinations and nightmares, experiences that make his everyday life "virtually unbearable."

To help Bill deal with these symptoms, Pax has been trained in extraordinary ways. Pax has been taught to warn Bill if people are standing behind him and responds to the command "block" to keep strangers from coming too close. If Bill becomes agitated or begins to relive memories of the bombings and explosions, Pax's quiet presence, unresponsive to any noises, makes him realize the dangers aren't real. Pax has been trained to remind Bill to take his medication and helps him stave off his nightmares. "In my dreams, I hear terrifying sounds of combat," he explains. "Explosions and gunfire that are so amazingly loud it feels as though they are right next to me. When this happens it causes me to bolt up, breathing hard, frantically looking around. Then I see Pax. He's calmly lying on his pillow sleeping. If there was an explosion or gunshot, Pax wouldn't be lying down. I know instantly it was all in my mind and I begin to calm. Before, it would take me much longer to gain control of myself. It's a small thing, but an amazing gift to me." Pax has helped Bill be able to leave his home and interact with others, whose conversation is focused more comfortably on Pax, easing his sense of profound isolation.

Like Dace, Pax was trained by a prisoner, Laurie Kellogg, who is serving time for murdering her husband who she says abused her for many years. Although Laurie had never met Bill, she felt a deep connection to him because they both are PTSD survivors. Pax was the first puppy she trained for PBB for a veteran returning from Iraq, but years of domestic violence allowed her to understand Bill's symptoms and what skills Pax needed to learn to assist him. "Pax gave me a chance to deal with some of my PTSD symptoms and opportunities to grow and get stronger," Laurie says. "In turn Pax learned to help Bill deal with his PTSD symptoms. Pax made me feel normal and alive again. He gave me freedom inside this prison. It isn't the fences or the bars or walls; it is what you build up around yourself. So Bill is still in a type of prison and I hope Pax can give Bill freedom within his prison."

Their journey together has not always been easy, and Bill is quick to admit that working with Pax was stressful at first.

Pax's barking would startle Bill and magnify his symptoms, so Bill had to retrain Pax not to bark. Recently, Bill has remarried, and he now feels more present with his three children and his wife in ways he never imagined, and he attributes this to Pax. Pax has changed two lives. A veteran and a prisoner both have found freedom from their traumas because of a loving, gentle, soul, a young yellow Labrador Retriever, Pax bringing peace to two lives.

There are 61 million veterans and their families in the United States who could potentially benefit from a psychiatric service dog. They are an ever-increasing population living with extraordinary challenges. As Raymond's and Bill's stories show, the lives of emotionally wounded veterans can be dramatically improved by working with a trained psychiatric service dog. And I encourage readers to refer to the Resources section at the end of the book to learn more about these services.

4
Sit, Stay, Soothe: Training Your New Companion

Once you have selected the dog that seems perfect for you, you are ready to explore your training options together. There are numerous books and resources available that outline general techniques for training your dog to follow basic commands, but dogs who will become PSDs must have additional training that is unique to the disabilities of their partners. Unlike with guide dogs, for example, who all tend to undergo similar training, PSDs are trained to mitigate the effect of the disabilities of individuals with wide-ranging types of emotional issues. This training is quite specialized and is not often available in many service dog training programs.

If you have adopted your dog from an established PSD program, your dog will already be highly capable of performing many tasks, although you may discover that with additional training together you will learn how to gain the most benefit from your partnership. In most cases, however, you will have adopted your dog on your own and will need to work with a trainer who can help you and your new dog learn training basics, as well as the more specialized tasks that you will need your PSD to perform. In either case, the goal is to work with a trainer who is ethical, non-judgmental, knowledgeable about mental health disabilities, and highly skilled in basic training and task training techniques.

In recent years, two organizations that specialize in providing PSDs to military veterans have established extensive training programs for these dogs and their handlers. Although the programs are limited to veterans, they can provide a useful model for the types of training that might benefit all PSDs. The dogs in the Puppies Behind Bars (PBB) program are bought as puppies directly from reputable breeders or are bred for the job by selected PBB breeders. At approximately 8 weeks of age, the puppies are assigned to the inmates who will be their caretakers for the next 18 months. The puppies share a cell with the inmates in a designated housing area of the prison, and receive daily massages and approximately three hours daily supervised "puppy play" time outdoors, weather permitting. The focus of training at that early stage is on bonding, housebreaking, and teaching the puppy its name.

After the puppies have spent a few days bonding with the inmates, the more specialized training begins with basic commands, such as sit, stay, come, heel, and watch me, with each dog progressing at its own pace. The dog then graduates to more advanced tasks, including retrievals, opening and closing doors, and turning on and off lights. Finally, the dog is taught complicated skills that involve a sequence of linked tasks such as hold, bring, and give. At approximately 6 months, each puppy is transferred for one month to another facility to be paired with a different inmate of the opposite sex, allowing the pups to get used to being handled by multiple people of both genders and to respond to the commands of another person. The inmates work together as a team, providing support and encouragement to each other's puppies. After 12 months, depending upon the skill level and maturation of each individual dog, the puppies are taught specialized commands that will be used in working with wounded warriors with PTSD or TBI.

Finally, the dog is introduced to its prospective handler and the dog and the veteran go through a two-week intensive training period together. This process of customization to the specific requirements of the human partner and the living situation (in an apartment with elevators, a home with children, and so on) is critical to the long-term success of the match. When they have finished, the teams receive certification at a PBB graduation ceremony. PBB does an in-home follow-up visit after six weeks, a recertification visit after one year, and yearly visits to check on the training process and the dog's health, and to recertify the veteran and the dog as a working team.

The first veteran to receive a PSD through the PBB program was helpful in identifying the opportunities and challenges of the program. Bill (from Chapter 3), emphasized that for him it was critical that his support system be present during the two-week training process. Because Bill's PTSD symptoms were so severe that he could barely leave the house even to run errands, just flying to attend the two week training program was a huge undertaking, and his distress was intensified by spending so much of the training process in public. Bill relied on his wife to provide the support and comfort he needed to cope with the many new situations he was facing, and his experience has helped program coordinators be more sensitive to the specific needs of veterans with PTSD.

Bill recalls an incident that occurred a few days after meeting his PSD, Pax, before they had completely bonded or he had been fully trained to go out in public alone with her. Bill, Pax, and his wife had stopped at a restaurant at the Air Force Academy to have lunch, but when they approached the counter to order their meals, they were told that the dog was not allowed in the facility. As the confrontation ensued, Bill experienced an increased level of anxiety as his breathing grew much more rapid and he became physically shaky. "Appearing calm on the outside while inside the world is unraveling to the point where you just can't take it," he recalls. A few days later, at the end of an exhausting day of training for Bill and Pax they entered a hospital with his trainer, who "pushed me beyond my breaking point. This is the problem with having an invisible injury." I rushed out leaving my trainer behind wondering what went wrong. Outside I was so shaken, I could not speak. Fortunately my wife was there and knew me well enough to tell my trainer to just leave me be for a while." Thanks to Bill's efforts, the restaurant ultimately changed its policies and PBB trainers were made more aware of the effects of PTSD and how to prepare their candidates for these types of altercations, which often confront individuals with invisible disabilities. Gloria shared that, "learning from Bill's feedback, in December 2008 PBB stopped sub-contracting its two-week 'team training' out to other service dog agencies. PBB conducts all of the training in-house, with instructors who have decades of experience working with people with psychiatric disabilities."

The NEADS program has also learned to anticipate the challenging situations many veterans with PSDs will face. NEADS puppies are donated or purchased from various reputable breeders and then, from eight weeks old until 16 weeks old, live at the Early Learning Center (ELC), where they are socialized and learn basic commands. At approximately 16 weeks, the puppies are then matched with an inmate or a foster family to continue the training process. With the help of a trainer, the prisoners work with their canine partner five days a week, 24 hours a day. On the weekends, pups are taken out of the prison to be exposed to the outside world, where they attend concerts, go to restaurants and stores, enter airports and railroad stations, are introduced to crowds, and are familiarized with any environment they might encounter in their working life as service dogs. On a weekly basis, the dogs are exposed to different sights, sounds, and smells that they may encounter with their human partner while a NEADS trainer works with the prisoners to introduce the dogs to a growing vocabulary of commands.

At approximately 16 to 18 months old, the pups are transferred to the NEADS training center in Central Massachusetts for further task training. At the conclusion of this extensive training process, the canines know more than 70 commands and are ready to be brought together with their veteran handlers. During a two-week training period, as the pup and the handler bond, the handler works with the trainer to learn the commands and how to react to different situations, sounds, encounters, and so on, and the handlers are taught to exercise their partners each day to keep the dogs strong and healthy. After graduation, the NEADS staff checks in on the dog and its partner after their first two weeks on their own, while at six and 10 weeks the partners provide a written report of their progress. A survey is completed on a yearly basis and the teams are retested every two years.

Raymond, who was partnered with Dace, recalls that his experience with the NEADS program prepared him for many of the obstacles he encountered. Raymond was impressed with how well trained Dace was and the number of commands she knew fluently, but observes that NEADS recommends that he integrate even less-frequently needed commands into his routine so that's Dace's early training is reinforced. Raymond has been able to continue training Dace to assist him by implementing the positive training techniques he learned at NEADS and has taught Dace to "find the pill bottles" and other additional tasks. Raymond felt less prepared for how his wife and children would react to a dog that was not a pet, but that had been trained specifically to help him with his disability, a topic we'll look at in great detail in an upcoming chapter. For example, Raymond was told that family members should avoid giving Dace treats, though the temptation always exists. It is difficult to prepare for every situation, but Raymond benefits from the information he received from the NEADS staff and their ongoing support and advice.

Although Raymond and Bill benefitted from programs that trained their PSDs specifically to their individual needs, it is more likely that you will learn how to train your own PSD through self-training and training with a qualified, knowledgeable, positive trainer. The term *dog trainer* is not completely accurate here because the dog trainer is actually training the handler as well as the dog and must be equipped with excellent communication skills, knowledge of body language and other subtle cues, flexibility, and empathy. The first step in this process is to find an experienced trainer who understands your disability and the specific tasks your dog will be expected to perform. You may have already selected a trainer who has assisted you in the selection of your PSD. The trainer also needs to understand how your disability might impact the training process. For the sake of both the handler and the dog, who both may be survivors of trauma, a trainer who appears overly controlling, domineering, or hostile should be avoided.

Though dog training techniques and philosophies vary, I strongly recommend a trainer who follows a positive training approach. Positive reinforcement training focuses on rewarding the dog's actions and behaviors in such a way that encourages the dog to no longer perform unwanted behaviors in favor of performing the behaviors that are desired. Aversive tools like shock collars, pinch collars, and other such tools can be especially problematic in the case of those with disabilities who may be unaware of how their physical movements may affect their PSDs and could actually work to undermine the trust between the handler and the dog. Training a dog can represent a huge time commitment and can be a financially and emotionally extensive journey without any guarantees. A loving and respectful bond is essential if the dog and the individual are to work in partnership to overcome the obstacles ahead.

The trainer should also be able to work closely with your counselor or psychotherapist to gain insights into your unique situation that will allow him or her to best collaborate with you and your PSD in the training process. Micky and Nancy, whom we met in Chapter 2, are both experienced dog trainers who were capable of training their own PSDs, but Tracy and Celia needed to work closely with trainers who could recognize their particular needs. Tracy's disability impacted her ability to focus at times and she struggled with retaining information. She needed to keep her training sessions short, with constant positive reinforcement, for her as well as the dog. Tracy also struggled with communicating clearly with others due to her high level of social anxiety, which in turn presented difficulties with learning how to communicate with her dogs. Tracy's trainer taught her a two-way communication technique that allowed her to read her dog's body language, cues, and feedback so they could communicate better with each other. Throughout the process, Tracy's trainer had to be patient, clear, supportive, and constantly reinforce the techniques and cues necessary to allow her to work successfully with her dog.

Due to shifts in moods and capabilities, Tracy, like others, had trouble dependably keeping a regular training schedule. If she was feeling upset, angry, or anxious, she knew she would not work effectively, and even possibly undermine the previous training. Tracy also needed to work with a trainer who understood that her disability might at times interfere with the scheduled training appointments. If Tracy experienced mood shifts or felt angry or irritable, her trainer would halt the process so that Tracy never took her frustrations out on her dog. In such cases, the dog and the handler can pick up together later when the handler's emotional well-being, patience, and focus are restored. A trainer needs to understand that such bumps in the road are common, unintentional on the handler's part, and must simply be accommodated.

Throughout this process an experienced trainer not only needs to know how to read the handler's body language, but also the dog's. The trainer must know how to praise at the right times to reduce pressure and stress, pace the training to both the handler and dog's abilities, and be consistent. This takes a highly skilled trainer who can adapt to each individual handler's moods while acknowledging that every dog also has a unique temperament, personality, and training needs.

Foundational training is absolutely essential in order for a dog to be properly prepared and successful in the higher-level training that is required of a PSD. The handler should begin the training process by enrolling the dog in basic obedience classes that instill appropriate manners, as well as taking the dog out on frequent "field trips" to places where dogs are allowed, to expose the PSD in training to anything and everything it would encounter in the outside world in the future. Such things would include people of all shapes, colors, sizes, and ages, as well as other kinds of animals; vehicles of all types and descriptions; objects that hang, flap, or float in the air, such as balloons or flags; a variety of strange noises; different surfaces like stairs and elevated walkways; and exposure to such extremes as fire and water at ground level, to name only a few such obstacles. A handler needs to use his or her imagination in trying to predict what the dog might encounter in the course of its work and anticipate how the dog might react in those situations. The dog must be able to follow basic commands in the face of many distractions, and I recommend that this first phase of training end in the dog successfully passing the Canine Good Citizen test administered by a registered tester (which can be located on the AKC Website *www. Akc.com*).

After you and your PSD in training have developed a high proficiency with basic skills and have passed the Canine Good Citizen test, you are ready to start working with a trainer (if you have not already selected one) on specific task training as well as what many refer to as public access training. The tasks that a PSD might need to know range widely, just as the symptoms of a psychiatric condition can vary considerably, and what is a useful task for one person might be totally useless for another. It is essential that the tasks directly mitigate the effects of the disability of the individual. A good place to start when deciding on what tasks your dog needs to know is to identify what things you have difficulty doing yourself due to your disability and to brainstorm with your trainer how your dog can assist in those areas. Examples of some of the tasks that PSDs have been trained to perform include: offering counterbalancing or bracing for those that have medication side effects that can cause a fall; turning on lights and searching when the team enters a residence; interrupting negative or self-harming behaviors and redirecting the handler; providing a tactile alert for an individual with Dissociative Identity Disorder to assist him or her back to a functional state; and identifying for a person if what he or she is seeing is real or a hallucination by having the dog do a visual check of the surroundings and alerting if it finds anything out of the ordinary. In addition to the many ways that the PSD can assist its handler at home, it may also play a major role in the individual's ability to interact with others in the community and be able to function at work.

Micky has trained Jake specifically to help in those areas of her life where she needs the most assistance. Without him, simple things like going food shopping or to school and work would not have been possible, because a good part of Micky's anxiety manifested itself as disabling physical ailments, ranging from searing back pain and sciatica to migraines and asthma, as well as anorexia that left her light-headed and weak. Jake was trained to wear packs that toted Micky's stuff around when she could barely straighten up, let alone carry a purse or briefcase, and learned to flawlessly navigate the crowded streets and narrow aisles of NYC stores without a mishap. He became skilled at bracing himself when she needed physical support, pressing his head and neck against her when she needed psychological support, and towing her along safely when blinding headaches left her exhausted and disoriented. His extensive vocabulary included directives like Slow, Hurry, Steady, Go Ahead, Left, Right, Back Up, Forward, Turn Around, and Serpentine.

After the dog has received basic training, public access training involves the handler and the PSDIT, at times with the trainer, going out into public places to learn how to handle all different types of everyday situations appropriately. It is important to note that, at this time, your dog is not a fully trained PSD, but a Service Dog in Training (SDIT). Laws differ by state whether a SDIT is given the same access in public places as fully trained service dogs, and certain requirements may need to be met before a service dog in training is allowed (see Resources pages 235-236 for where to locate state laws).

If you live in a state that does not allow SDIT public access, training can still take place in parking lots, and pet and feed stores, as well as public events where pet dogs are allowed, especially outside toy stores and malls where dogs can get lots of exposure to kids, as well as to many other distractions like traffic, moving shopping carts, car horns, and car doors slamming; at hotels that allow pets (to practice using elevators, stairs, and raised walkways); and in outdoor, open-air flea markets and farmer's markets (if pets are allowed). For a list of ideas for socialization see the "Puppy Socialization Checklist" at *www. k9events.com.*

In order for your dog to be adequately prepared for public access, your dog should be able to pass the Assistance Dogs International Public Access Test (PAT at *www.adionline.org/publicaccess.html*) or a derivative test based on the PAT, which can be administered by your trainer. During the test, your dog will be required to successfully demonstrate its ability to work in a busy and crowded public environment. You can prepare for the PAT by ensuring that your dog is completely proficient in its foundational skills and has had plenty of "hands-on" experience being out in public in a variety of environments for at least six month to a year. Some of the skills to practice include:

- ~ Going under tables and ladders, into revolving doors, through metal doors, or over objects.
- ~ Taking your dog on every type of moving transportation which includes buses, subways, cars, ferries, walking on the moving walkways at airports, and so on. It is, however, not advisable to use escalators with your service dog, as it is just too easy for a dog's nails, toes, or pads to become pinched n the escalator and cause severe damage.

- Exposing your dog to a wide range of sounds, including congested traffic, car horns, buses and trucks, sirens and alarms, fire trucks, loud machinery, road construction, crowds shouting or cheering, children playing, video games and other computer sounds, and other sources of banging, grinding, drilling, grating, and alarms.

- Exposing your dog to people of every type and physical description, from people wearing hats and holding umbrellas, to those wearing mustaches and beards, to individuals with different cultural backgrounds and languages and even eccentric behaviors—everything that this team might run into.

- Making sure your dog does not react to being tugged, pulled, or touched or respond to verbal attention or commands from strangers who, intentionally or otherwise, may attempt to manipulate your PSD inappropriately.

The list of possible distractions is endless, and caution should be taken not to overexpose the dog or handler during the training, but to take the process slowly and ensure that both are coping well before moving forward and increasing the stimuli.

Preparation is essential so that you feel capable of coping with whatever challenges arise in the public environment. For instance, exposing the dog to every type of flooring, whether creaky wood, stone, grates, heavy tiles, and so on, is critical, as are training the dog to go to the bathroom anywhere when grass is not available and being prepared to clean up after the dog no matter the environment. Learn to expect the unexpected. If you plan to be out for an extended period of time, you may want a collapsible water bowl to allow your dog a drink. If you find yourself in a small public restroom, will your dog be able to fit into the tiny stall with you, or will it wait outside the door of the stall? What if your equipment or leash breaks while you are out? You may want to carry with you a lightweight leash/collar combo that is commonly used on show dogs, which is small and light yet works very well as an emergency measure. Dogs sometimes become ill and you need to have some kind of a plan of what to do if that should occur. You can either take the day off or, if you have a backup dog, he or she can fill in until your other dog recovers. Some people find that a friend, relative, or partner can temporarily be a service person for them and assist them until their PSD is ready to return to work.

The dog must also be prepared to respond in public to the unique behaviors of its handler, such as the onset of feelings of anxiety, irritation, or even a dissociative state. This is where the handler's therapist can assist the trainer to learn how to read the handler's symptoms, such as a change in breathing, a flushing complexion, eyes glazing over, freezing in place, and other signs that the trainer must be alerted to so he or she can adapt the training process. The therapist can role-play ways to cope with situations that might trigger the handler's symptoms and brainstorm about what tasks the dog can learn to prevent or mitigate the effect of these symptoms.

Completion of the CGC or the PAT is not mandated for public access, but federal law does require that a service dog be trained to work or perform tasks to assist its disabled handler and not be a direct threat to the safety or health of others.

Such tests provide assurance to the handler that the dog is in fact ready to work in public and the certificates provide valid proof of the dog's abilities if ever needed in the future. However, federal law does not require certification of fully trained service dogs, and they are not required to have any special tags or certifications, or wear vests or other special equipment when out in public.

From time to time, you may be challenged by employees of business establishments who are familiar with the use of guide dogs but not the use of PSDs by people with invisible disabilities. Preparation and role-playing are essential so that you will feel comfortable and confident entering restaurants, movie theaters, places of employment, and other public places with your dog but, if confronted, you should not feel compelled to provide personal information about yourself or state the nature of your disability. Doing so may only be confusing and cause difficulty for others with PSDs. The only questions you are required to answer are whether or not you are disabled (though you do not need to provide the particulars about your disability), if your dog is a pet or a service dog, and what your PSD is task trained to do, though you do not need to provide a lengthy and detailed response and certainly not one that violates your privacy about your medical condition (*www.ada.gov/svcanimb.htm* and *www.ada.gov/qasrvc.htm*).

To help you protect your rights in these situations, I recommend that you have quick access to records documenting the training you and your dog have received, certificates or awards earned, up-to-date licenses, and your dog's current medical and vaccination information, whether it's kept in the glove compartment of your car, a file, or your office. You may also want to carry a pre-printed card that summarizes the laws regarding the use of PSDs in public places in your wallet or in your PSD's vest pocket (see Appendix 1 for sample documents). Although not legally required, these documents can give you confidence in the event of a confrontation, while at the same time educating the public about your rights as a disabled handler.

Keep in mind, however, that there may be times when such a confrontation is just not advisable and you may want to pursue your goal at another time, with the help of others, or through such means as writing letters to the staff and management of places where your access was challenged. By sharing the difficulties, struggles, and obstacles that you face with other individuals with PSDs you can gain insights in what and how to prepare for your own training needs (see the Resource section for a list of Yahoo groups that focus on service dogs, service dog training, and service dog laws) and work together to educate others about the role of PSDs in public places.

As you embark on your training together, you, your trainer, your therapist, and even your canine partner will find many opportunities for your PSD to assist you both at home and in public, sometimes in ways that you never imagined. Based on deep emotional bonds and a respectful professional relationship, the training process itself can be quite empowering, as you gain confidence skill, and commit to the care of another living creature. For many, participating in the dog's growth from a puppy or young adult into a fully trained service dog is deeply therapeutic, enriching, and rewarding.

5

A Member of the Family: Helping Everyone Get Along

For many individuals, a PSD can be an empowering companion, a source of strength, courage, self-confidence, and insight, a catalyst to a fuller and more independent life. Working with a PSD, however, requires an enormous commitment, not only on the part of the handler, but also for those closest to him or her, and, as with any new introduction into the family, you can expect a period of adaptation and adjustment. Good preparation, along with lots of information and patience, can help you and your family members, relatives, and friends adjust as you take this life-changing step.

One of the most common difficulties surrounding the introduction of a PSD into the home is the need to reinforce the understanding that a PSD is a working dog and not simply a talented family pet. When Bill received Pax from the Puppies Behind Bars program, his counselors stressed that, in order to strengthen and maintain Bill's relationship with Pax, it was important that his children refrain from petting and playing with the dog. Not surprisingly, his kids were heartbroken that the fun-loving Labrador Retriever was off limits, and after consulting with PBB, Bill and his wife decided to introduce another dog into the family for his kids to play with.

Bill and his wife soon found a young black Labrador mix named Max, whose family was concerned that he was not getting proper care and exercise while they were at work all day. When Max and Pax first met, they played well together, but within a few days Max became overbearing and aggressive. It soon became clear that Pax was stressed by Max's arrival. Because Bill and his wife recognized that Bill's relationship with Pax was the priority, Max was returned to his previous home.

Bill and his family were disappointed, but were willing to see if a different dog might be the answer when they found Maggie, a young Whippet mix, wandering in a parking lot less than a week later. Maggie appeared emaciated and filthy, but very friendly, and without encouragement she leaped into their car. Bill and his wife searched unsuccessfully for Maggie's family, and she very quickly adapted to her new home. It was clear that Maggie had previous training and knew all of her basic commands and, unlike Max, Maggie was calm, easy-going, sensitive, and sweet. Pax's and Maggie's temperaments were complementary, and they soon became the best of friends, wrestling and playing ball together. Maggie is now Pax's playmate, helping to provide him with plenty of opportunities for exercise, while the children have a family pet and are able to respect the special working relationship Pax has with their father.

Raymond's family, also, had to adjust to the introduction of a PSD into their lives. Raymond's wife, Sarah, supported him throughout his recovery and his decision to adopt a PSD, but she had no experience with dogs and she was unaware of Dace's basic daily needs. Raymond's two children were thrilled that Dace was joining the family, but everyone soon struggled with "figuring out the lines between service dog and pet." Especially at holiday gatherings, it was difficult for Raymond's relatives to refrain from giving Dace treats and to think of him as a working dog, not a pet. The NEADS staff helped Raymond educate his family about Dace's role as a PSD and develop a daily routine that has helped them support this distinction.

But bringing Dace into their lives had some unexpected consequences for Sarah and Raymond as well. When they fought, Dace would nudge and try to separate them, his behavior becoming a distraction that often reduced the tension of their arguments. Dace's presence seemed to help Sarah and Raymond learn how to communicate better, to avoid the yelling that often accompanied their fights. Through time, however, Dace allowed Raymond to become more confident and he began to realize that a feeling of dependence lay at the heart of his relationship with Sarah. Raymond's lifelong dream was to be a public speaker, and Dace provided him with both courage and a cause as he began advocating for veterans by speaking publicly about his healing journey with a PSD and the NEADS organization. Dace had empowered Raymond to live more independently, while helping convince Sarah that his needs could be met without her. Eventually, Raymond and Sarah amicably agreed to divorce.

Micky, too, experienced serious difficulties with her family once Jake was fully trained and began accompanying her in public. For most of her life, Micky had viewed new or novel situations with dread, but Jake took on any new challenge with enthusiasm. Now, there were lots of questions when she went out in public with Jake, but Micky was always in "educator mode," cheerfully chatting with anyone who asked about Jake and how he assisted her. Whenever they went out together, Micky's mother hated the attention and the emphasis it placed on Micky's tumultuous emotional life. For Micky, leaving Jake at home was non-negotiable, so little by little she and her mother saw less of each other. There would be no healing of their relationship until her mother acknowledged the emotional trauma Micky had experienced in childhood.

With Jake in tow, Micky dared to attend Al-Anon meetings, where once the thought of entering a room filled with strangers would have left her gasping for air. Jake facilitated Micky's first trusting relationship with a therapist, giving her the confidence to speak, allowing her to breathe and pace herself instead of being overwhelmed and unable to continue. Therapy helped Micky to see that her relationship with her significant other was based on codependence, and to recognize his drinking for what it was: alcoholism. With the help of her Al-Anon friends, her therapist, and Jake, Micky gathered the strength and courage to leave her toxic relationship and feel safe enough to live alone again.

As these stories reveal, the introduction of a PSD into relationships and family life with long-established patterns can sometimes interrupt the status quo. How can you and your family share the responsibilities of having a PSD without blurring the boundaries? Will your children understand the role of a PSD? Will your partner be jealous or no longer feel needed? How will you explain the role of a PSD to your extended family, and what reactions can you expect? Can you take family trips with your PSD? What impact will the PSD have on your family pets? Who should take care of your PSD if you become ill or your routine is temporarily changed? As you and your family come to learn all of the ways that a PSD can improve your lives, there are many factors to consider.

Introducing Your PSD to Your Family

Change, no matter how beneficial, can be the source of stress. Talk openly and often about the challenges of introducing a PSD into your family's life. Begin the dialogue before you adopt a PSD and continue to explore how everyone involved adapts and adjusts after the dog is trained and in the home. Talk to others who have adopted PSDs about their experiences. Take advantage of the resources noted in the Resources section of this book. Your therapist and trainer may be able to provide insights and suggestions as new issues emerge. If possible, find a therapist who has previously worked with service dogs and can provide support, strategies, and assistance to you and your family, especially during the critical adjustment period. Working collaboratively with your trainer, therapist, and the members of your "inner circle" can best ensure a successful outcome.

The introduction of a PSD into your household may force family and friends to face your hidden disability; this, in turn, may cause them discomfort, embarrassment, or feelings of shame. Many people with PSDs are surprised when their family members and friends are hesitant to be seen in public with them while they are working with their PSDs. Open up a dialogue. Be direct. Would they be as reluctant if the dog was offering you physical support? Is their discomfort due to the high visibility of the dog or interruptions by the curious or uninformed? Are they concerned about the stigma of mental illness? Discuss these issues with your therapist. Use message boards, blogs, and Web groups to exchange information and brainstorm with other PSD handlers about strategies for dealing with reluctant family and friends. Try taking short frequent outings at first, over time your family and friends may gain a level of comfort with your PSD. In some cases, conflicts about the presence of a PSD can cause such dissension that the handler must decide whether or not to cut the ties to those individuals who aren't willing to accept their disability.

A handler's growing reliance on a PSD may make some family members, particularly spouses, feel less needed. This is where family therapy can be instrumental in opening up a dialogue about resentments and any other issues that family members might have been wrestling with due to the presence of the PSD. The therapist can help these individuals discover the positives that the PSD is bringing into their lives and identify the benefits to the disabled family member. In addition, a therapist can discuss how they can utilize the spare time they now have available to them, and how they can reduce the feelings of loss and diminished need. The handler's new freedom can open up doors of opportunity or it can expose patterns of dependence.

PSDs and children

Your PSD's relationship with you, the handler, is an essential component of predictable and reliable teamwork. Young children can unintentionally distract and confuse the dog; older kids can feel left out and deliberately undermine the training process. It is advisable to plan ahead so your school-age kids understand that your PSD is a working service dog with responsibilities and rules to guide its behavior. It is so important that they be "on board" and not encourage the dog to misbehave. Impress upon them that the dog is required to do certain things a certain way for a very good reason: your health, safety, and welfare!

Ask your trainer to include your children in the training process, coaching them about interactions that are appropriate as well as the limitations of certain situations. Exposing kids to the training process will help them understand that this dog is not a pet, but has important work to do. Depending on their age and ability to take direction, children can help reinforce appropriate behaviors and participate in training set-ups and role-playing. Most kids like playing tracking, retrieving, and find-it games, which will help reinforce the skills the handler needs the PSD to perform.

It may be difficult for some kids to live with a dog that is not their pet. At some point, after the PSD has settled into a stable routine, you may consider adopting another dog as a pet. You can also channel their caregiver instincts by allowing them to adopt other pets like fish, reptiles, gerbils, and other small mammals that they can care for in their rooms. This may help them avoid interacting inappropriately with your PSD. Additionally, if the child is old enough, he or she can volunteer at the local animal shelter, walk neighbors' dogs, or join a 4–H club and work with handling animals.

Other pets

If you have other animals living at home, it's important that your PSD and your existing pets get along. The presence of other animals can excite the PSD to stalk or pounce, while the stress of being hunted can adversely affect the health of your other pets. Dogs, cats, birds, small mammals, and pocket pets can also interfere with the PSD's ability to focus and respond to the handler. The PSD must be comfortable in the presence of other animals; family pets cannot distract or lure the dog away from its work.

All introductions should be made while the PSD (and other animals, as appropriate) are on leash, and begin at a distance. All appropriate behavior should be rewarded, and without raising your voice at the PSD or at the other pets. If the PSD becomes highly stimulated or overly agitated, increase the distance between the PSD and the other pet. Try again after the dog regains its composure. Until the PSD's behavior around the family pets is reliable and predictable, the dog should not be left unsupervised.

It's best to introduce your PSD to the family dog in a neutral space, not the home. It's a two-person job. If possible, have your trainer walk the new dog alongside you while you walk the pet dog. At first, keep the dogs at a distance, walk parallel to each other, and chat informally so the situation looks and sounds amiable to both dogs. If the dogs' body language signals that they're feeling comfortable in each other's presence, then walk the dogs closer to each other. Always remain below threshold, taking it slowly until both dogs seem relaxed, curious, and ready to sniff each other. If the meeting has been successful, walk toward your home and ask the trainer to stay a while before you are left alone with the dogs. Use a crate, pen, or baby gate to keep the dogs apart when you cannot supervise them.

If problems remain after repeated attempts to socialize your PSD with your current pets, you may need to make some adjustments. Try segregating the pets or setting up areas that are "off limits" to each animal. If the PSD is unable to control its impulse to chase or pounce on any of the family pets, or does not seem comfortable around them after several days/weeks, then the potential PSD might not be an appropriate candidate, or you may have to consider finding new homes for any pets that cannot adjust. This may be difficult, depending on the pets' age, habits, and personality, and each family member should be given the opportunity to speak on behalf of the best interests of existing family pets. Remember that part of choosing the right dog should be whether it can get along well with everyone living in the home.

Dogs who are already family pets can prove to be unsuitable for work as a PSD because their age, temperament, relationships with other family members, and/or current habits preclude them from switching gears from pet to service dog. However, in some instances, the pet dog is already very attached to the potential handler. Some families have no problem "giving up" the dog to its new role and supporting the rules that come with it. Even in such cases, however, it may be difficult for those who have a relationship with your pet to change the way they relate to him/her. Once again, it is recommended that you utilize the services of a counselor to smooth the way.

When Tracy decided to adopt a second PSD, she was apprehensive about how the semi-retired Baron might react toward the new dog, Finola. Tracy worried that Baron would feel replaced or abandoned, and the dog picked up on her negative emotions. Tracy worked with her therapist to overcome her feelings of guilt and discussed her fears of being unable to provide Baron with the time and commitment she had given to him before Finola entered their lives. She explored ways to manage provided the two dogs with enough care, walks, playtime, compassion, and love. Her trainer suggested giving the dogs separate rooms and stressed the need to keep the dogs at a respectable distance, until they both indicated they were feeling more comfortable with each other. Eventually, through the recommendations she received from her trainer and the support she received from her therapist, Tracy was able to work through the mixture of complicated emotions she was experiencing. Now, Tracy, the retiree, and the new PSD enjoy a sense of tranquility and joy in sharing their home together. Baron and Finola are now the best of buddies, sleeping together on the bed with Tracy, both alerting her when necessary. And yes, they play together, too! Time, patience, and training helped these two dogs gain confidence and be at ease with each other.

Daily Life With Your PSD

A service dog is a professional who has daily responsibilities; you must keep its skills sharp by practicing the right way, everyday, in order to maintain their ADA compliant skills and routines. Tracy's dogs follow a routine that includes making sure she takes her medication and gets up to go to work. Micky relies on Jake to get to work and school, and to use public transportation, so strict adherence to his training protocols is essential, lest she forfeit her public access rights.

As your PSD enters your family's life and routines, the specific do's and don'ts of how family members should interact with your PSD will depend solely on how the behavior affects the dog's ability to work. Like people, some dogs are better at multitasking then others. Some PSDs can play with the children in the house or backyard one minute without it interfering with their ability to respond to their handler's needs the next; other dogs need to remain in close proximity to their handlers at all times. If you received your dog from a program, you will likely have received instructions designed to maintain the dog's skills and training at acceptable levels long term. If you have trained your own service dog, then it will be up to you to be alert to situations that could cause possible training issues or erode skills, and deal with them accordingly.

When the PSD comes home, I recommend that, at least initially, most of the caretaking be done by the handler. Feeding, walking, and grooming, as well as time spent reinforcing training, petting, and cuddling, help to build a positive bond between the handler and the PSD based on mutual respect and trust. Once the bond is secure, other family members can slowly step in and begin to assist with the dog's care. If this attention from others interferes with the dog's ability to respond quickly and appropriately to the handler, the handler must resume full care of the PSD. But if the PSD continues to work effectively, then family members, especially children, will benefit from and enjoy working with you in caring for and reinforcing the training of the PSD.

A PSD's training is based on following rules, and family members should behave consistently. To avoid confusion, you should establish firm guidelines for:

- ~ Where is the dog allowed to be at mealtimes?
- ~ Will the dog be allowed on furniture?
- ~ Will there be "off limits" areas for the dog?
- ~ Will there be prohibited activities, like tug-of-war games and play fighting?
- ~ Can the PSD run off to romp at will, or will you use formal "release" and "report" directives?
- ~ How are treats earned, and who can give them to the dog?
- ~ Who is allowed to walk the PSD?
- ~ What are the circumstances under which family and friends are allowed to give the dog affection?

How strictly you and your family follow the rules depends on how your dog continues to perform its service. Should a handler elect to become a little lax at home, he or she alone suffers the consequence. But poor behavior or an inability to respond appropriately in public is another issue entirely, one that may cost the handler his or her protected status under the ADA.

Like all dogs, PSDs welcome affection, perhaps even more so because their training is based on positive rewards. Most PSDs are selected for their ability to be physically close; they welcome intense handling (petting, hugging, and cuddling). When at work, the affection is as genuine as the "pat, pat, pat" for a job well done. When off duty, affection can come from family, friends, and even strangers out in public in various ways and forms. However, be careful that family members' affectionate interactions with your service dog don't come at a cost, like giving table scraps to the dog during family meal time. The desire to express affection for your dog should be redirected in a way that does not undermine the dog's skills or routines. If anyone in your household begins to lose patience, yells, or abuses the dog, the dog's safety must come first. The dog should be removed immediately from the situation and, if needed, professional help should be sought to protect the animal.

Outside of your home, plan ahead of time how you will handle large family gatherings, holidays, and, most importantly, public outings to restaurants, museums, the theater, and so on. What things can you do in advance to make it easier for all involved? Call ahead; tell the maitre'd or inform security that you will be accompanied by your PSD so that the establishment can prepare in advance of your arrival if necessary. Carry the equivalent of a doggie diaper bag (contents: a bowl, a pad to lie on, wipes, treats, a chewy or a toy) with you, so you can tend to your dog without imposing.

When considering bringing the dog to a private home, confirm in advance that your PSD is welcome. Though the ADA states that service dogs are allowed in public places, it does not extend to churches, private clubs, and homes, so permission to attend with your PSD is essential. Some family members and hosts just don't want a dog in their homes; knowing this beforehand will prevent conflict. Some handlers decide not to attend family gatherings due to the lack of accommodation; others suggest that their own homes be the site for the holiday and family gatherings. You should consider how long the gathering will last and how you will meet your dog's needs during that time period. You may choose to leave your PSD behind to attend a private social gathering where it would be more of a hindrance than a help if the dog came along. In such instances, you could rely on a "service person" to assist you.

Family and friends may be unprepared for the confrontations that sometimes arise with those who are unaware of the laws relating to PSDs. To help answer any of these questions, you may want to keep a card with information about the federal and state laws quickly available in the dog's vest pocket. A good source for access information is from the U.S. Department of Justice titled Commonly Asked Questions about Service Animals in Places Of Business (*www.ada.gov*). Ask supportive family members to role play these scenarios at home with you so that you are practiced at diffusing the situation as quickly and effectively as possible. Inform them that you are capable of coping with these situations yourself and they will not have to step in to assist you.

All PSDs should be given ample non-working time to relax As the dog's handler, you need to teach the dog to differentiate between working, being on call, and being off duty. You can reinforce such distinctions through directives and signals, with a change of equipment (such as taking off the dog's service vest), or by changing location. To relax, Bill's PSD, Pax, rough-houses with Maggie, the family dog, while Jake goes for walks in Prospect Park, where he swims in the lake and plays with the local kids.

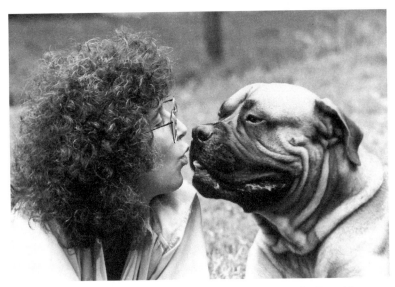

Micky and Jake having a moment in Prospect Park, Brooklyn.

Even when some dogs are off duty, they remain attuned to their handlers and their needs; Nancy's dog, Windy, is always ready to alert Nancy of an oncoming panic attack, even when they are engaging in dog sports. There is no single prescription for relaxation, as long as the dog's playtime activities don't affect its ability to work. We'll look in the next chapter at other techniques that can help alleviate the stresses that service dogs face.

There may also be occasions when you must leave your PSD behind. Some vacation destinations may just not be suitable for dogs, or you may need to consider the people you are traveling with. Some require quarantine or immunizations that would not be appropriate. International trips by air can be quite daunting for even the most seasoned travelers; traveling with a dog might be a deal-breaker.

You should consider who will care for your PSD if you are sick or hospitalized, or in the event of some other emergency. Hospitals must allow you to have your PSD, but you will need the assistance of friends and relatives to help you with the walking and feeding of your PSD, because staff members are not legally responsible. If the dog cannot be with you in the hospital, then a designated caregiver will need to fill in until you are available. Whether it's a professional pet sitter, your dog trainer, or a friend, this individual needs to be responsible for feeding, walking, maintaining training, and providing companionship to your PSD in your absence. The PSD should be wearing a service dog tag that lists an emergency phone number and your veterinarian's telephone number (see Appendix 1). Keep a list of your PSD's dietary needs and make sure you have given your consent for your veterinarian to care for the dog in your absence.

You may also need to make plans in case your PSD gets sick or injured. You may be able to take the day off from work and spend the time with your PSD for a short period of time, but if illness or injury requires a lengthy recuperation, there will be a major disruption in your daily routine. You should plan ahead for assistance with the tasks your PSD ordinarily helps you perform. There are occasions when a friend or family member may be asked to step in and provide a special form of care. Dace, Raymond's PSD, had an ear infection that required medication. Because Dace disliked the procedure, Raymond asked his wife to administer the offending ear drops, thereby preserving the trusting relationship between Raymond and his PSD.

To be prepared in the case of family emergencies, you should make sure you have easy access to your records. When you acquire your dog, all program paperwork, bill of sale, adoption or AKC registration papers, dog license, microchip registry, CGC certifications, and so forth, should be registered in the name of the handler. If your family pet has become your service dog, arrange to have any paperwork, including veterinary records, changed or transferred to reflect that you are the handler. Legally your dog falls into the same category as a medical device and cannot be taken away from you by another family member or if you and your partner divorce. To prevent future problems, your attorney can draw up a contract that stipulates that your PSD is a "service dog" and is the property of the "disabled" handler. I also recommend that you include a provision in your will for the care of your dog in the event of your death.

No matter how much preparation you have, learning to adjust to life with a PSD requires a great deal of patience and compassion, as Michele and her husband discovered over the course of their relationship. A year after Michele adopted her dog, Mordecai, she moved in with her boyfriend, Robin and got engaged to him the following summer. At first, Michele's fiancé was skeptical about Mordecai's role. He didn't like taking the dog with them everywhere the couple went and saw him as an unnecessary crutch, an obstacle to Michele's healing and independence. But one day while the couple was arguing, Mordecai was able to calm her down by pawing her gently and Robin finally recognized Mordecai's abilities to soothe Michele's fears. As their wedding day approached, the couple fought about Mordecai's attendance at the wedding, but in the end a friend took care of him during the ceremony and Mordecai stayed with Michele's parents that night. The next day, after the honeymoon, Michele was thrilled to have Mordecai back at her side.

For Robin, having a dog cohabitating within the confines of the house, and sharing the bed and couch with the couple were significant issues. "Nothing in my life experience has prepared me for having a dog that is treated like a human being," he recalls. "Michele talks to Mordecai as if he can understand English. This was a MAJOR life decision dropped into our relationship without my input." Michele feels Robin sometimes resents and is jealous of Mordecai, but he has also come to have his own strong bond with the dog. Michele described getting upset in couples therapy, when Mordecai started nudging and pawing her, helping to reduce her level of stress. Moments later, Mordecai came to Robin's side, now nudging and pawing him as well, and it dawned on Robin that Mordecai was there for him too.

Through time, Robin has become much more comfortable going out in public with Mordecai and Michele, and stands up for them when they are challenged. "Michele has shown a perseverance and enthusiasm in figuring out the laws and rules pertaining to Mordecai," Robin remarks. "She keeps printouts of several applicable statutes that she takes along with her as well as all the various tags and cards for Mordecai. Whenever she is confronted, Michele always remembers that she serves not just herself but is also a public face for all service animal teams. I am so very proud of how she handles this. In the time that Michele and Mordecai have been working together, I have seen that at least a score of businesses that we frequent have changed their policies from some variation of 'No animals except seeing eye dogs allowed' to some variant of 'service animals only.'"

Today, with the help of her "two men," Robin and Mordecai, Michele "leads a fuller more normal life." Mordecai has also helped improve and strengthen Michele and Robin's relationship by acting as a catalyst to healthier communication. If they are fighting, he will continue to nudge and paw at them until they speak to each other in a calmer manner. Mordecai, it seems, is not only Michele's psychiatric service dog, but he has taken on the role as the couple's marriage counselor as well. For Michele and Robin, Mordecai has helped them live a more balanced life as they enjoy walks, relax, watch a movie or television, read books, or just spend time cuddling together.

As we have seen, many PSD handlers find the help of a therapist, trainer, or PSD program essential when facing the concerns of friends and relations. Consider joining a local or

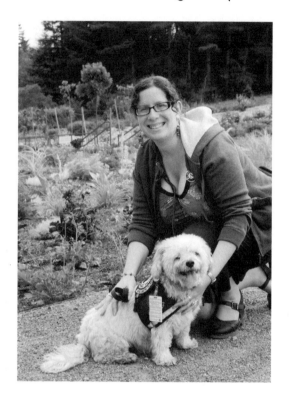

As an Americorps member Michele was performing outreach at the Humboldt Botanical Gardens with the assistance of Mordecai. He has provided Michele with the ability to maintain a full-time job.

online PSD support group (see Resources section page 234) as a way to meet people and gain a wealth of information from some of the most experienced sources. Some hold events that include doggie playtime, fundraisers, and opportunities to share recommendations with other handlers and their PSDs. If a group does not exist in your area, consider starting one. It is critical that all family members have the opportunity to voice their feelings while exploring ways to cope with the changes that a PSD brings to everyone's lives.

6

Dogs Have Issues, Too: Helping Your Dog Cope With Stress

It takes a very special dog to be a Psychiatric Service Dog (PSD). In order to be effective, the dog needs to be in tune with its handler's mental state, mood shifts, environment, and practical needs, but it can't be so intuitive that these concerns continually impact the dog in a negative way. Because the handler may be suffering from stress-related difficulties, a dog that is too empathic or intuitive may also begin to show signs of increased stress. As we saw earlier, when Tracy adopted her first PSD, Baron, her deep depression affected him so adversely that she had to give him a sabbatical from work. Perhaps more than any other type of service dog, PSDs must have a balanced life filled with time for work, play, and relaxation.

The emotional well-being of PSDs is not just a practical concern, but an ethical one as well, but consistent ethical standards have not always been adequately developed. Clearly the impact of assistance work on the dog's emotional and physical well-being is an area of scientific research that needs to be explored. Animal behaviorist Alan Beck points out that, although service dogs are trained to help, "their utility to people must not include psychological or physical abuse, and whatever discomfort is absolutely necessary is clearly balanced with benefits that will foster improved health for both the human and the animals involved." Beck specifically addresses considerations surrounding service dogs in the following three areas:

1. Source of the animals.
2. Work stress for the animal.
3. The well-being of the animal after his or her usefulness is over.

Beck and others believe that many of the stresses service dogs face could probably be avoided if trainers and handlers were better educated and trained in how to work with service dogs in ways that helped to avoid physical and mental stress. In this chapter, we'll turn our attention from the handler to the dogs themselves and explore some of the strategies that can help ensure the dog's emotional and physical health and well-being.

Let's begin by looking at language. Terminology referring to the relationship between the handler and dog should convey mutuality, integrity, and respect. *Handler* or *partner* is preferable to the terms *owner* or *master,* which convey overtones of power and control. In addition, handlers and partners should not be seen as "using" their PSDs to perform service tasks; their relationship is a human-animal bond that flows in two directions. Although some also see the term *handler* as implying dominance, it is used in this book with the highest regard for a balanced relationship between humans and their PSDs. Another problematic term is *replacement dog* when referring to a PSD's successor. PSD tasks can be learned, but each dog is special and the partnership can't be duplicated. Many programs prefer *successor dog* as a preferable and more humane term when a committed, trusted, beloved PSD is to be retired or dies.

Sensitivity to the language we use has helped raise awareness about our relationships with animals, as have public policy and legislation. In 1965, the British Parliament took one of the first steps toward consistent ethical standards when it created the Brambell Commission, which embodied the minimum standards for animal welfare in its "Five Freedoms":

1. Ensure your pet is free from hunger, thirst, and malnutrition.
2. Ensure your pet is free from discomfort.
3. Ensure your pet is free from pain, injury, and disease.
4. Ensure your pet is free to express normal behavior.
5. Ensure your pet is free from fear and distress.

Expanding on these freedoms as a standard of care for your PSD's welfare means being aware of the PSD's need for quality nutrition and adequate water, comfortable shelter, enough space, veterinary care, grooming, exercise, playtime, downtime, the alleviation of stress, companionship, and love. At every stage of the handler/PSD relationship, the physical and emotional needs of the dog must also be met, and no harm or abuse should ever be permitted.

To ensure the animal's basic health and safety, a new handler would benefit from enrolling in a canine first aid class available through one of a number of the organizations providing courses. Two highly recommended sources are the Red Cross (see *www.redcross.org* for their "Dog First Aid" information) and Pet Tech (*www.pettech.net*) programs. PSD handlers should carry at all times a canine first aid kit they either purchase or make themselves, as well as the phone numbers of their regular veterinarian and the local emergency animal hospital. In times of crisis these precautions can be lifesavers. Tracy's PSD Finola wears an ID tag that identifies her as a service dog and provides her contact information, emergency contact number, her veterinarian's number and Finola's microchip number (see Appendix 1).

In choosing a veterinarian, you should look for one with previous experience providing healthcare to service dogs. Networking with other service dog handlers in your area, or asking your trainer, therapist, and friends for referrals can be helpful in finding the right healthcare provider. It is highly recommended that handlers meet with the veterinarian in advance of a medical crisis to explain how your service dog mitigates the effects of your disability. With this information the veterinarian can meet your needs and reassure you that you can make an appointment quickly if a crisis arises, because without your PSD you may not be able to function or go to work. It's important that your vet and his or her staff respect your relationship with your PSD and provide care to both of you as a team.

There are numerous resources available to help cover the cost of care to service dog teams with financial needs. In some cases, a veterinarian may provide discounts or may have specifically set aside funds to cover the costs. Other organizations, like the International Association of Assistance Dog Partners (IAADP), can help service dog handlers receive discounts from some providers. You may want to consider pet insurance plans, some of which may provide discounts for service dogs. You also may be eligible for the Social Security PASS program, which facilitates your ability to work, or you may receive a benefit from a flexible health spending plan or be able to deduct the costs of caring for a service animal as a medical expense on your taxes (check with your CPA). (See the Resources section, pages 247-248 for more information about these resources.)

Another vital aspect of your PSD's health and well-being is quality nutrition and weight management. In addition to heeding your vet's recommendations, you may want to consult a canine nutritionist or visit one of the Yahoo canine nutrition sites to get further information pertaining to your PSD's specific needs, and twice a year *The Whole Dog Journal* lists its choices of top-quality dog foods. With the help of a canine nutritionist, you might opt to cook nutritionally balanced meals or feed raw. The bottom line is that the diet must be balanced and of high quality. A PSD handler must also be responsible for grooming his or her service dog. Many people have found the tasks of grooming their dogs and brushing their teeth provide structure and routines that help them take better care of themselves as well. Tracy shared that, when she gives Baron and Finola their medications, she is reminded to take her own. She is committed to keeping her PSDs healthy, clean, emotionally and physically well by providing them with the best of care, accompanied by love and respect. Given how much you rely on your PSD, you want to take strong preventative measure to ensure lifelong good health.

Exercise is essential for all dogs for both physical and emotional well-being. Individual dogs require different levels of exercise, which may change over the course of the dog's lifetime. Mindy and Celia, and Ninna and Scout all benefited from the long walks they took together. Others have enjoyed taking classes that focus on a canine sport such as Agility, Rally, C-Wags, Canine Freestyle, and so forth that suit the dog's needs and temperament. Nancy discovered that Agility classes helped Windy, a very high energy dog, remain focused, calm, and more balanced when working. These sports can be fun for the team while also reinforcing maneuvers that the dog needs to practice. For example, a dog that has learned Canine Freestyle will be trained to work well on both sides of the handler, back up, heel, and perform other behaviors that are necessary when out in public. One dog might love Agility and another might prefer Canine Freestyle, while others are stressed by the competitions and classes. Handlers must learn how to read their own PSD's stress signals and body language to access accurately what is best for their dogs, but these fun sports can be a wonderful way for handlers to bond with their dogs while getting out and meeting other participants.

Every service dog has different needs regarding balancing work time, down time, exercise, and relaxation. Windy required intense and frequent exercise whereas Baron and Jake benefited from romping outside, spending time sniffing, rolling in nasty things, being couch potatoes, and just being dogs.

Dogs, like people, need time off from work, whether it be to play, hike, or just relax. Michele and Mordecai take walks in the redwoods and romp on the beach for some outdoor recreation, or Mordecai plays with their cats in the backyard and enjoys chewing on his ragged stuffed bunny to expend some restless energy. Michele has become friends with two other service dog handlers in her area, and the three of them take their dogs for on- and off-duty outings around town together. This allows the dogs to have some fun socializing and gives the women time to talk about service dog issues, training, and life.

A wonderful video displayed on the Canine Companions for Independence Website (*www.cci.org*) shows a service dog one minute capably assisting its handler, a veteran with a prosthetic leg, and the next, after its service vest is removed, running in the yard as only a dog can. Even though at times it is amazing to watch PSDs work and see the skills they are able to perform, handlers must always remember that their service dogs are living, breathing, sentient beings with various needs requiring the best quality of care at all times.

A core component of a healthy relationship between handler and PSD is the dialogue and communication they have developed through time with one another. In order to attain this, the handler must become educated about canine body language, and stress and calming signals pertaining specifically to his or her own PSD (A list of excellent resources is provided in the Resources section, pages 243-249). Just like humans, not all dogs communicate in the same ways. Some dogs bark when stressed; others may lick their lips, pant, shake, and so on. A PSD is aware of the handler's emotional and physical state, and needs the handler to be attuned to this knowledge in return. Learning to read your PSD's behaviors ensures that you can respond appropriately to your dog's needs and fosters a bond based on mutual respect.

Like humans, dogs respond to the demands placed on them by their environments with symptoms of physiological stress. Long-term and/or persistent exposure to stress hormones, specifically Cortisol and Norepinephrine, can weaken the dog's immune system. Although dogs may respond to stress differently, some general indicators of stress include persistent yawning, licking, sniffing, scratching, chewing/licking oneself, panting, more frequent urination, bowel changes, diarrhea, vomiting, pacing, changes in communication patterns seen through posture, head and eye movements, shaking, sweating paws, salivating, sudden shedding, changes in appetite, or level of energy, and so on. Some of these behaviors may be due to a medical issue so the first step whenever you notice any change is to rule out any physical ailments. If your vet finds no physical ailments, you may need to try to determine the causes of your dog's distress and alleviate these conditions. One of the most common sources of stress for dogs is any change in their daily routine or environment. Has your dog been "working" more recently, or getting more, or less, activity than usual? Has he or she had more exposure to crowds in public places or to new people in your life? Have you changed his or her diet, or your daily schedule, or taken the dog to unfamiliar places? Even changes in the weather or introducing new objects, routines, or household products into his or her environment can cause your dog stress. Try to identify if you have made any changes in the dog's routine or environment that may be causing stress and begin by eliminating these triggers.

There are also a number of stress-reduction techniques that you can try. The PBB program provides daily massages for the puppies in its programs to help them bond with their handlers and get used to being touched by their partners, veterinarians, and others. NEADS integrates stress-reduction techniques, like giving the dogs a day off and ensuring there is downtime and playtime, into programs educating handlers on the basic needs of their PSDs. These programs emphasize that the health and welfare of their PSDs are priorities that must be maintained on a daily basis.

As a Reiki practitioner, a QiGong (an ancient Chinese meditative martial art form) Instructor, and a certified canine massage therapist, I teach all of my clients stress-reduction and relaxation techniques they can use with their PSDs. There are a number of techniques such as "Tellington Ttouch," "Healing Touch For Animals," deep breathing, meditation, visualization, and yoga that you can practice with your dog, which you might want to explore on your own or with a group of handlers in your area. Tracy relates that, when she is practicing QiGong with her dogs together and lying beside her, both her breathing and her dogs' breathing slow down, and the experience helps her to release some of her own anxiety and experience profound feelings of love. You might also seek out the services of trained professionals who can assist with techniques to decrease the PSD's stress, including herbologists, homeopaths, acupuncturists, bach flower remedy specialists, behavioral consultants, and holistic veterinarians and some trainers.

No matter how much you work to eliminate stress in your PSD's environment, there will be times when your dog simply needs "a day off." As a PSD handler, have you prepared for how you will manage your routine if your PSD is sick, is recovering from illness or surgery, seems overly tired or stressed, and so on? Have you asked your friends, relatives, and others to assist you if your PSD is not able to work for a brief period of time? Have you discussed with your employer that you will need to take sick days off if your PSD can't work?

Although it's not an option for everyone some handlers, like Tracy, have trained two PSDs so that one can have a day off while the other one goes to work. Tracy has found that because Baron is older and less active, he is a good partner for activities that are more relaxed, like going to the movies or accompanying her to restaurants, where he lies at her feet and nudges her when he senses her anxiety level is rising. In contrast, Finola has much more energy and is better suited to going to more active places like the grocery stores, museums, malls, and so on. By being aware of her dogs own talents and needs, Tracy diminishes stressful situations for all of them. Micky has now worked with several dogs and has learned that if she adopts and begins training a new dog as one of her PSDs is entering mid-life, the younger dog is ready to take over when its time for the older PSD to retire.

These are some of the issues you should consider in ensuring that your dog enjoys a healthy, productive, and happy life. As PSDs and other service dogs have become more common, the Assistance Dog International has taken the lead in establishing general guidelines for "Standards and Ethics Regarding Dogs" that would benefit all service dog organizations and their members. Their policies state:

"Standards and Ethics Regarding Dogs: ADI also believes that any dog the member organizations train to become an Assistance Dog has a right to a quality life. Therefore, the ethical use of an Assistance Dog must incorporate the following criteria.

- An Assistance Dog must be temperamentally screened for emotional soundness and working ability.
- An Assistance Dog must be physically screened for the highest degree of good health and physical soundness.
- An Assistance Dog must be technically and analytically trained for maximum control and for the specialized tasks he/she is asked to perform.
- An Assistance Dog must be trained using humane training methods providing for the physical and emotional safety of the dog.
- An Assistance Dog must be permitted to learn at his/her own individual pace and not be placed in service before reaching adequate physical and emotional maturity.
- An Assistance Dog must be matched to best suit the client's needs, abilities and lifestyle.

- ~ An Assistance Dog must be placed with a client able to interact with him/her.
- ~ An Assistance Dog must be placed with a client able to provide for the dog's emotional, physical and financial needs.
- ~ An Assistance Dog must be placed with a client able to provide a stable and secure living environment.
- ~ An Assistance Dog must be placed with a client who expresses a desire for increased independence and/or an improvement in the quality of his/her life through the use of an Assistance Dog.
- ~ An ADI member organization will accept responsibility for its dogs in the event of a graduate's death or incapacity to provide proper care.
- ~ An ADI member organization will not train, place, or certify dogs with any aggressive behavior.
- ~ An assistance dog may not be trained in any way for guard or protection duty. Non-aggressive barking as a trained behavior will be acceptable in appropriate situations."

There are minimum standards for Assistance Dog Partners, courtesy of Assistance Dogs International. The assistance dog partners will agree to the following partner responsibilities:

1. Treat the dog with appreciation and respect.
2. Practice obedience regularly.
3. Practice the dog's skills regularly.
4. Maintain the dog's proper behavior in public and at home.
5. Carry proper identification and be aware of all applicable laws pertaining to assistance dogs.
6. Keep the dog well groomed and well cared for.
7. Practice preventative health care for the dog.
8. Obtain annual health checks and vaccinations for the dog.
9. Abide by all leash and license laws.
10. Follow the training program's requirements for progress reports and medical evaluations.
11. Arrange for the prompt clean up of dog's waste.

The ADI, as one of the leading "accrediting bodies" for service dog programs, also sets useful standards for the behavior of Assistance Dogs in Public (see: "Public Standards" *www.assistancedogsinternational.org*), Minimum Standards for Assistance Dog Partners (see "Dog Partner Standards" at *www.assistancedogsinternational.org*), as does the Delta Society with their Minimum Standards for Service Dogs. (See *www.DeltaSociety.org*.)

By following these standards, all organizations and handlers can be assured of providing the quality care that allows

PSDs to perform their necessary tasks while meeting their own needs for a healthy and compassionate environment. For their valuable service, companionship, devotion, and love, all PSDs deserve this much and so much more!

7
The Golden Years: Knowing When to Hang Up the Leash

Every individual who decides to embark on this healing journey with a PSD is aware that these living creatures will one day grow older. For some, the realization will eventually come that their companions can no longer perform their usual service; for others, a dog's failing health signals a greater decline that even with foresight and preparation can be heartbreaking. This possibility should be explored before you take on the responsibility of sharing a life with a PSD.

Even for those who have given these considerations careful thought, however, these circumstances can be difficult when they actually arise. As your dog ages, you should watch for signs that your PSD is slowing down, having greater difficulty with mobility, is less interested in going to work, eating, going for walks, and experiencing discomfort with fluctuations in temperature, all indications that it might be time to consider your dog's retirement. Discuss your aging dog's needs with your veterinarian, therapist, and trainer, as well as the services that your dog provides for you. In some cases, you may want to consider training a new dog before your PSD's health begins to decline. If this option isn't feasible, can you turn to a service person for assistance, take time off from work, or change your routine to accommodate your PSD's diminished capabilities? After all the years that your PSD has assisted you, you'll want to plan ahead so your dog can age gracefully, with respect, comfort, and compassion. In this chapter, we'll look at how others have handled this process and review some of the practices and resources that can help everyone move through this inevitable transition.

~

Due to the effects of the severe childhood abuse that Mindy had survived, she had never allowed anyone to get too close to her. She always kept others at a distance and protected herself from anyone who might harm her, disappoint her, or let her down. When Mindy adopted Ninna, she never dreamt that they would become so close and how deep their mutual trust would become. Ninna saw parts of Mindy no one else had ever seen, and Mindy let her into her world with cautious arms. Within time, Mindy's days revolved around Ninna, providing her with a structure and routine, allowing her to live a more balanced life than she had ever previously achieved. Ninna was Mindy's rock, and Ninna relied on Mindy for her food, walks, shelter, and care. A new world had opened for Mindy when she and Ninna learned how to manage life together.

When Mindy adopted Ninna, she was approximately 5 years old. Just a few years later, Ninna started having severe coughing fits, and Mindy was devastated when the veterinarian informed her that Ninna had congestive heart failure. Mindy then took her to a cardiac specialist and began to explore holistic healing methods to help manage Ninna's symptoms. She put Ninna on a low-sodium diet to maintain a low body weight and started her on medication to decrease the coughing symptoms. With this healthful regimen, Ninna was not experiencing any symptoms of heart failure other than a heart murmur detected by the veterinarians, and her coughing was alleviated by the medication.

It was Mindy who suffered the most from her dog's diagnosis. She had not contemplated living without Ninna, and the potentially fatal condition forced her to face a reality she wanted to deny. But Ninna was definitely not ready to die; she was still filled with curiosity, sniffing everything on the ground during her walks, garbage picking, and hiking with Mindy for miles. During this crisis, Mindy learned that she needed to focus on how strong, stoic, and filled with life Ninna remained despite her condition.

Fortunately, Ninna survived for seven more years in good health and then, when she was 15 years old, she started to decline. She began to exhibit symptoms of severe arthritis and had difficulty walking. When Ninna's kidneys began to fail, she was no longer interested in eating, seemed to be losing her sense of smell and vision, and started falling over, moving very slowly and looking completely disoriented. After weeks of hoping that Ninna would find peace on her own, Mindy realized that she needed to help her beloved PSD die. Mindy knew this was the gift she had to give Ninna after everything Ninna had given her. Mindy was able to find a vet who would come to her home to euthanize Ninna, and Mindy and her therapist discussed every detail of the day for which the procedure was planned to help Mindy prepare for the loss. She asked that her therapist be present to support her and she began to make plans for after Ninna was gone. Mindy felt that having structure would help get her through the days ahead on her own.

Mindy and a friend went out that morning and bought Ninna a pizza, and together with Mindy's therapist they all ate some of it together at home. Ninna stopped eating when the veterinarian's arrived, almost as if she knew, Mindy recalls, and was lying comfortably on her bed with Mindy's friend and her therapist. Mindy took some photographs of Ninna and then spent some time saying goodbye to her. When the vet started the procedure, it seemed as though Ninna was gone before the injection even entered her bloodstream. Ninna had died so calmly and peacefully, Mindy was convinced that she was ready to let go. Still, Mindy wept with grief and, after Ninna's body was removed, Mindy left her apartment to spend a couple of days at her friend's house.

After 10 years together with Ninna, Mindy struggled to regain her bearings and cope with the loneliness she now felt in her life. Before Ninna's death, Mindy had received a full scholarship to enter a graduate program in library science, conducted primarily via the Internet, and after Ninna was gone she immediately began to dive into a new routine as a student. When her rent increased a couple of months later, she decided to move out of the apartment that she and Ninna had shared. She knew moving before Ninna died would have been too difficult an adjustment for Ninna.

As Ninna started to decline, Mindy had thought that adopting another dog as her PSD would not have been the right choice for them. A year later, although she misses Ninna, Mindy is still not ready for another dog. With intensive graduate study, Mindy is aware she doesn't have the time yet to devote to building a relationship with another dog, but Mindy has relied on friends and her therapist for support. Ninna's ashes are still being stored in Mindy's therapist's office until she is ready to take them home, but it is reassuring to her that they are safe and protected. Mindy still struggles with loneliness and the lack of Ninna's comfort, love, and companionship while working to re-establish her daily routine. Through her relationship with Ninna, Mindy experienced bonds of love she hadn't imagined and a depth of pain she never wanted to endure, but Mindy now is able to smile rather then cry when she thinks of Ninna, her beloved healing companion.

Celia, too, experienced the decline of her trusted PSD Scout. After 10 years together with Celia, at age 14, Scout began to exhibit difficulties with her mobility and was diagnosed with bad hips. Celia respected Scout's increased inability to navigate her way through the New York traffic and crowded streets, and she began to take Scout to work less frequently with her. At the same time, Celia got a new job closer to where she lived so she was able to go home during the day to walk Scout. Celia felt that adapting to the new work environment would be too stressful for Scout and she came to the realization that "it was the natural time for Scout to retire." Fortunately, her job provided her with the flexibility to take time off to care for Scout.

A few nights before New Year's, Celia took Scout to the dog run for exercise, where another dog slammed into her violently.

Scout seemed fine when she first arrived home, but shortly after she started to fall over. Celia asked a friend to drive them to the emergency veterinarian, and by the time they arrived Scout was paralyzed from her neck down. After two days at the hospital, Scout was not improving, and Celia knew that it was time to help her die. The next day was New Year's Eve and Celia felt that the most caring, respectful way she could conclude the year was by celebrating Scout's life.

When Celia entered the ER on New Year's Eve day with all of the foods that she knew were unhealthy for Scout, she describes how Scout "gobbled up the food and then died happy and peaceful." Though Celia knew that Scout was ready to die, they had shared 10 intimate years together, and recovery from Scout's passing was difficult. Celia mourned privately and it took Celia quite a while before she was ready to scatter her ashes in the woods.

Nine months before Scout died, Celia had adopted ARLO!, the exclamation point of his name accurately capturing the level of his exuberance. Celia had been persuaded by friends to get another dog because they were concerned how she would cope once the aging Scout was gone. Celia had been quite resistant to the thought of another dog, but with much coaxing she ended up at the shelter and met the irresistible shepherd cattle dog mix she renamed ARLO! He was a handful, and Celia struggled with finding the time to train and bond with him while she was dealing with Scout's declining health. Now, while Celia was grieving Scout's death, ARLO!'s presence provided added stress. Training ARLO! would be a major project under the best of circumstances, and Celia's trainer felt the undertaking would be too great given Celia's grief, but she was stubborn and, although ARLO! would ultimately not become a service dog, he is now a wonderful companion that shares life at home with Celia.

Celia's fiancé, Walter, was a major support for her through the grieving process. Celia and Walter are now married and this relationship has helped Celia with her disability. Soon after Scout's death, Celia was offered a job in Texas, far from the city that is filled with memories of her life with Scout, where ARLO! has room to run. Celia, Walter, and ARLO! have all adjusted to a new life together, but Scout will always be with Celia in her heart, that one special dog that changed her life forever.

Bullmastiffs have a short life span, eight to 10 years at best, so when Micky saw that Jake was having difficulty getting in and out of the car, she knew it was time to plan Jake's retirement. She started by cutting back on his activities: no more classes, or obedience trials. She also decided it was time to start looking for his successor. Using the same plan that had worked so well with Jake, the search began, and not too long after, Jody, a pretty red bullmastiff joined the family. Jake seemed to love the new addition as much as Micky did.

At about 9 years of age, Micky stopped taking Jake to work with her. It was becoming increasingly difficult for Jake to stand up; he was getting stiff and arthritic. Jake stopped using the stairs after he tripped and fell on the way up to the bedroom. He needed more and more assistance in moving his stiff body from floor-pillow to sofa and back again. Jake was definitely suffering from "old." It was Jody's turn now, and she attended classed and went to work with Micky. She was not as effervescent as Jake, and Jody was easier to work with because she was more aloof with strangers and smaller in size.

On Memorial Day weekend, Jake was looking particularly awful; the light in his eye was fading. But the next morning was a real shocker; for the first time in his life, Jake had soiled his bedding. In total devastation, Micky called the vet, discussed Jake's condition, hung up, and waited for him to arrive. Meanwhile, Micky stroked Jake and held him so tightly she didn't know how she was going to let go. She couldn't stop thinking that she'd never put her arms around his wonderfully thick strong neck again. When the veterinarian arrived, Micky took a deep breath and looked Jake straight in the eye. It was time. She glanced away from Jake for just a moment, but when she looked back at him, Jake was already gone.

On that beautiful spring morning, life as Micky knew it came to a grinding halt. She was awash with grief. Nothing eased the pain. She couldn't speak, eat, or move. The migraines came in waves. Each breath was an effort. She was worn out, but not cried-out. The melancholy that surrounded her was suffocating. It was just Jody and Micky against the world. Yes, little Jody, service dog-in-training, was now suddenly thrust into the center of things, and she was glued to the side of the crumbling Micky. Jody was a full year younger than Jake was when he first "went public," and Jody was clearly grieving. So they started out conservatively, short trips and outings with a friend, Nancy, and her dog, Ben, who was Jody's best friend.

Slowly, Jody gained confidence and Micky's trust. In October, just four months after being pressed into service, Jody boarded an airplane to St. Louis so Micky could attend a Delta Society conference. Jody was relaxed and professional as she accompanied Micky throughout the conference center and during her presentation on emotional support dog training. The passing of the baton was seamless.

Micky planted an honor garden on her property where Jake's remains were buried. The gravesite has become a wonderfully soothing place. The flowers growing there are just as spectacular as he was; their dizzying fragrance fills the air. When she sits by his grave, the violence, turmoil, anger, and rage that consumed Micky seem like light years ago. Today, her life is as she always envisioned it while growing up: the earth mother, a little house, a kitchen garden, a field filled with flowers and animals—living in sync with nature.

~

Nancy, too, has been planning ahead. Although Windy is still alive and well, Nancy has thought long and hard how it may feel when Windy dies. Discovering Windy's abilities to allay panic episodes was utterly miraculous for Nancy, and Windy has been Nancy's virtual lifeline. Nancy struggles with imagining life without her precious Windy but knows the inevitable time will come. In the face of her fears, she has made a number of significant resolutions:

1. I treat each moment and day as if it's the last for her, and do everything possible to make her life balanced, healthy, and enjoyable. I strive not to overwork her— in fact, I have worked hard to deal with my condition so as to avoid Windy having to respond to my attacks and be seemingly always on the alert for them.

2. I have trained my two other dogs to perform the same tasks Windy does, and this enables Windy to get breaks

from her service dog work. I know when Windy is gone that they will be there for me.

3. I have resolved to try to remember the lessons Windy has taught me, and be thankful for them. I wish I could be more like her: forgiving no matter what, happy all the time, full of energy, and having a wonderful ego. She is able to focus when it's called for despite whatever else she may be doing, and when learning new things, will never quit until she understands what's expected. She's silly and fun in her natural state.

4. I will bury her with a ball, next to her pond here at home. Windy is obsessed with balls and water, and it will be comforting to know she's laid to rest in her favorite place with her favorite ball.

Nancy has trained two successor dogs, Breeze and Jingle, to be PSDs, with Windy's assistance through what Nancy describes as mentoring or role-playing. Breeze and Jingle follow Windy's lead and see her reactions to Nancy, and they mirror Windy's behaviors. Nancy knows that when Windy is gone, Breeze and Jingle will help her continue with a life that Windy first made possible for her.

~

As these stories reveal, there are many ways to think about the end of your PSD's life and service. For some people, as their PSDs near retirement age, it's useful to consider training another dog to not only help you navigate through your life but also to alleviate your eventual loss. Others may not feel ready to train their next PSD immediately but may discover new ways of mitigating their disabilities. After the deaths of their dogs, both

Mindy and Celia experienced major life changes, moved, started new jobs, and enrolled in school full-time. They both have struggled profoundly with adjusting to their new lives, but with the support of friends and environmental changes they are managing without a PSD, although they may choose this option again in the future.

Knowing when and how to help your dog die is one of the most difficult decisions you may face. In some cases, the dog may die peacefully in relatively little pain after a period of decline. In others, it may be clear that the animal is suffering and needs your help. Difficult as this decision may be to face, thinking about it ahead of time can make this event less stressful. Many people recall that they "just knew" it was time and felt as though their dog was telling them "I am ready." Some veterinarians will make home visits, and you should inquire well before you need it if your vet provides this service. Consider whether you will want emotional support during this period and, if so, ask a friend or your therapist if he or she can assist you when the time comes. Be aware that your empty house may cause you feelings of sadness and loneliness and whether you should make plans to have a friend stay with you or to stay elsewhere yourself for a brief period of time.

As Elizabeth Kubler-Ross has noted in her work, *On Death and Dying*, grief can include many stages of denial, bargaining, anger and guilt, depression, and resolve and acceptance, which ebb and flow throughout the grieving process. There are numerous Yahoo service dog groups and other support groups and hotlines that can provide you with support after the death of your PSD. (Ask your veterinarian for local resources or consult the Resources section, pages 249-250.)

For some people, rituals can be a helpful way to assuage grief and memorialize your PSD. A year after Ninna's death, Mindy posted an album on Facebook and heard from friends she hadn't been in touch with in years, a healing tribute to Ninna and the lives she and Mindy touched. Some find relief through doing art projects that memorialize their PSDs, writing a eulogy, poetry, a letter, or song, or creating a scrapbook or photo album. Others hold a ritual or ceremony that might include a memorial service, burial, spreading of ashes, a religious or spiritual ritual, returning to places that were shared, lighting a candle, making a charitable donation, or planting flowers, a tree, or a garden. Make sure to reach out to your support systems during this process and consider professional help if your grief is overwhelming.

I, too, have a story to share about the end of my journey with a very special dog. My story began with Umaya, who led me down a path that altered the direction of my personal and professional life. She opened a window into a world that I never would have imagined, one graced by educating others about the healing power of ordinary dogs to transform the lives of those with psychiatric disabilities. I owe this book and the journey I am on to her.

After surviving two bouts of cancer and radiation treatments with stoicism and strength, and a vicious attack by two dogs that nearly killed her, at almost 12 years of age Umaya started to fail. Although she had been undergoing holistic treatments and consumed a home-cooked diet, Umaya's body was deteriorating. She was having more and more difficulty walking, pottying, and, finally, eating. It seemed like once the heat of summer arrived, even with air conditioning, the changes in temperature were too much for her to handle. But Umaya was still filled with energy, wagging her tail, and seemed at times oblivious to her physical situation, so I continued providing her with hospice care as long as she seemed to have an acceptable quality of life. I am not sure if she was holding on to life for my sake or her own.

Her sense of smell was fading and, after years of making her organic home-cooked meals, I tried to entice her with liver, which she liked at first, but within a short amount of time stopped eating. I remembered from when she was receiving radiation that everyone would take their dogs out to Mc-Donalds after their treatments because all they could get their dogs to eat were Big Macs. After years of feeding Umaya the best of the best, I now routinely pulled up to the McDonalds drive-through window, where I requested just the patties for her, which she devoured on a daily basis. I guess it came down to whatever worked and she seemed happy. In the meantime, one year before Umaya died, Simcha entered our lives, another dark golden retriever filled with puppy energy and exuberance. I felt that Umaya knew that Simcha would be there to take care of me.

One night in September, I looked at Umaya and I knew that it was going to be her last night with me. She was almost 12 years old and I thanked her for all she had done for me. I told her I would find a way without her physical presence, but that she would always be with me and reassured her that it was time for her to let go. I held her for a while, but knew that she wouldn't go until I left the room. We shared our last goodbyes and I went to my bedroom and went to sleep.

At dawn, Simcha shot up out of bed whining and I knew at that moment Umaya had died. It took me a few hours to pull myself together before I headed into the living room to find Umaya lying there looking so peaceful, but no longer breathing. She had died quietly, while sleeping. I brought Simcha in to say goodbye, and a friend and I wrapped Umaya in a blanket. I called the vet and explained, with a sigh of relief, that Umaya had died peacefully. When we arrived at his office, my vet and several of his technicians and assistants met us in the parking lot, and we proceeded to carry Umaya inside. She was placed on the table and we cut some locks of her hair, and the staff made a paw print for me. We were all weeping. It was helpful to have some private time with her, and then my friend and I left to spend the rest of the day sitting at the lake where Umaya swam, grieving and struggling with knowing Umaya wouldn't be there to greet me when I returned home.

Umaya had touched so many people's lives that it seemed important to memorialize her together, and planning a memorial service gave me something to focus on to distract me from my grief. I decided to have the ceremony at Umaya's favorite swimming place where everyone would congregate in a circle and share their memories of her. A month later, more than 50 people—her vet, the vet techs, my clients, friends, family, Simcha, and so many others whose lives were touched by Umaya— attended the ceremony. Eulogies and stories about Umaya were read at the ceremony, and other rituals in her memory were videotaped so I could relive the event. If those who attended didn't feel able to read their own memories, others would read them for them, while others volunteered to read eulogies that had been mailed to me. It was a beautiful, breezy, sunny, autumn day when so many people celebrated Umaya's life and spirit and those she had touched were encircled by love and support. I also started a fund in her honor that provides veterinary care to those with service dogs who need financial assistance. Friends, family, and relatives make donations every year on my birthday, Umaya's birthday, her Yahrzeit (anniversary of the day she died), and holidays. The fund is an ongoing tribute to her providing care to service dogs in need (see the Dedication for where to make donations).

My friend Kathy's eulogy served as an eloquent memorial:

"My memories of Umaya rest in a number of particular images, which seem to capture both Umaya's spirit and the special symbiotic relationship between Umaya and Jane.

The first image is from puppyhood, one of the first times I accompanied Jane and Umaya on what unexpectedly turned out to be a great adventure. The season was early winter, the air was crisp, and we ended up at Lakeview Park in Lorain. I'm not certain if it was Umaya's first swim in Lake Erie, but it was an incredibly dramatic one. As Jane and I walked along the water's edge, Umaya ran ahead, bounded out the stone jetty, right off the end, breaking through the ice and plunging into the frigid waters. As terrifying as that moment was, I looked around and saw Jane flying down the beach and out the breakwall, with what looked like every intention of diving right into the lake after Umaya. I ran in their direction, positive that I, too, was going to have to dive in, and that would be the end of the three of us. By the time I was close enough to see clearly, Jane was poised precariously on the very edge of the stone, dragging a shivering and momentarily bewildered Umaya up out of Lake Erie by the collar. By the time I stopped screaming and shaking and crying, Jane and Umaya were playfully romping in an effort to reassure me that they were fine, and wasn't that an unexpected adventure?

Other joyful images fill my mind and my heart—of Jane and Umaya dancing to the music of the steel drums on the steps of Finney Chapel on Illumination Night, of Umaya rolling in ecstasy from side to side on a pile of beautiful autumn leaves, in a pristine snow bank, and on a decaying fish on the shore. What a nauseating ride home that was from Mentor Headlands. But I have to tell you that Umaya had a big smile on her face all the way.

What I remember most—the perpetual smile and wag, through the best of times and the worst of times. Never a complaint or a whine, seeing the joy in every day, finding every little wonder to wag about and refusing to surrender any of the fun of it all to the hard knocks of life. Umaya reflected the spirit embodied in one of Jane's favorite sayings: "Every day is a gift." I will remember this lesson, and am grateful.

Umaya's Eulogy

Many of you here are people who entered my life because Umaya introduced us or brought us together through her energy and wisdom. Because Umaya faced so many illnesses and physical challenges she connected me to a wide circle of animal healers in many places, and I feel blessed by knowing these people. I especially want to thank these remarkable healers—some present and some who can't be here today—who stood by both of us during her life and through her process of dying. These healers also cared about me and in some cases even inspired my own journey into new healing modalities or supported me to discover new dimensions in my lifelong goal of intertwining human and animal therapies.

Parallels between Umaya's life and mine made our shared relationship profound. Through these parallels in our physical and metaphysical lives, Umaya and I shared a powerful bond. What Umaya experienced as healing led me to follow her path in taking care of myself, and what I experienced as healing enabled me to lead Umaya on her path of recovery, but always our paths merged and we traveled our roads together. Because of our 12 intimate years together, Umaya and I shared so many life processes, trips, and discoveries that we formed a union of spirit and were able to communicate with each other.

Here are a few of the treasured memories in my Umaya album I'd like to visualize with you. You'll recognize many:

1. She would wag her tail, with her glow of "I'm alive" in the waiting room of my office after radiation, inspiring the whole room and bringing a smile to all of the people waiting for their psychotherapy appointments.

2. She always greeted people with a mouth full of her favorite toys and frequently would try to engage in a tug-of-war with her green snake toy.

3. Sometimes Umaya's gifted leadership seemed to start with an attention-getting behavior; many times during sessions with clients she would start licking the rug. This irritating behavior would however have exquisite timing since her ridiculous licking would distract us from getting too intense and permit us to regain perspective. This behavior also helped to identify that the individual was either feeling stressed or anxious. They frequently observed Umaya's behavior and recognized their own feelings.

4. *Watching Umaya swimming with such determination and strength. She glowed in the water.*

5. *When I played Bonnie Raitt or other music that had rhythm Umaya would leap up on me grasping my waist and we would dance together.*

6. *Her rolling in the autumn leaves with utter ecstasy elicited my playful sprit to join in and roll with her whether in leaves or snow when we would make snow angels together.*

Umaya's grace enabled many people to connect to her special wisdom. Their insights into Umaya's power touched me deeply because these people participated in and expanded our circle of special understanding. Umaya's brilliance and magnificent example taught so many of us how to get through our days—of suffering, of joy, of living, even of dying—with dignity and courage.

Umaya's process of dying amplified how she lived and helped us both reach closure with peace and grace. She lived each moment to the fullest—reinforcing for me the gifts of celebrating every day—and she died without struggle, peacefully in her sleep.

I'd like to have everyone now participate in honoring Umaya in two ways. First you'll float rose petals in the reservoir to symbolically preserve Umaya's healing spirit. After that you'll toss sticks and visualize her swimming to retrieve them as a way to liberate Umaya's energy into the elements. I will then spread some of Umaya's ashes into her favorite swimming place so now Umaya's legacy will and can live on within all of us.

Shalom
Jane Miller

Come Share In A Celebration of

UMAYA'S SPIRIT

(10/30/92 – 9/02/04)

1 PM Saturday, October 23
Morgan Street Reservoir (Rain location: Oberlin Inn, rear patio), Oberlin, OH

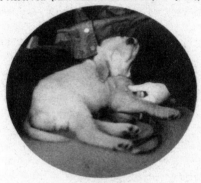

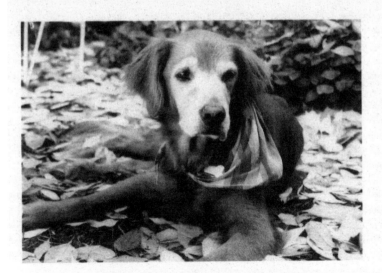

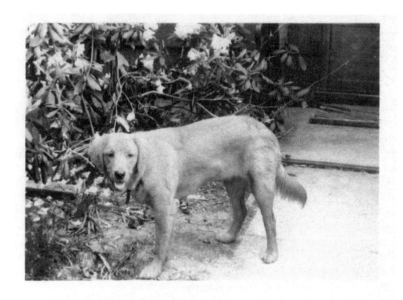

Please feel free to share memories about how Umaya touched your life.

If you cannot attend, and would like to contribute a story, send your words to jmiller@oberlin.net and they will be read at the tribute.

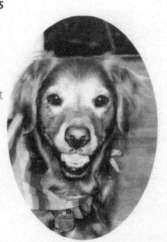

If you wish to make a donation in Umaya's honor please send it to:

Lakewood Animal Hospital,
Attn: THE UMAYA FUND,
14587 Madison Ave.,
Lakewood, Ohio 44107

The Umaya Fund will provide funds for pet owners with limited funds for paying their pet's healthcare.

Appendix 1
Sample Service Dog Cards

Have your ID card printed with your dog's photo and laminated.

OHIO Service Dog SD

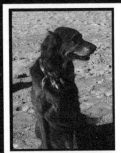

Jane Doe
123 Niceplace St.
Anywhere, Ohio
44444

Champ - Golden Retriever
Chip ID - XXX-XXX-XXX

Service animals are legally defined
(Americans With Disablities Act, 1990)
and are trained to meet the
disability-related needs of their
handlers who have disabilities.
Federal laws protect the rights of
individuals with disabilities to be
accompanied by their service animals
in public places.
Service animals are not considered "pets."

Sample Service Dog Emergency Preparedness Card

Reg. AKC = SN 80988101 AVID is 045-092-286
Handler: **Tracy Corso**
Dog: "Baron," a Labrador Retriever; yellow, N male
THIS DOG IS MEDICALLY NECESSARY.
DO NOT SEPARATE FROM HANDLER.
In case of emergency, contact:
Jane: 1-800-457-0345
Vet Contact: Dr. Barney: 216-226-0400

Sample Card Outlining Your Legal Rights

Federal laws which protect individuals with disabilities include the ADA; the Fair Housing Amendments Act (1988); Sect. 504 of the Rehabilitation Act (1973); the Air Carrier Access Act (1986/90); and other regulations. The person who is accompanied by the service animal is responsible for its stewardship (behavior, care, and well-being), must obey animal welfare laws (such as leash, cruelty, or other similar regulations), and is liable for any damage done by the service animal. About service dogs, contact the Delta Society National Service Dog Center at (425) 266-7357. About the ADA, contact the U.S. Department of Justice ADA Information Line (800) 514-0301 (V); (800) 514-0383 (TDD).

Laws that protect the rights of people with disabilities who have service animals

The Americans with Disabilities Act (ADA, Title III. 28 CFR 36.104) defines a service animal as any animal that is individually trained to perform tasks to assist a person with a disability. The specific nature of the person's disability may not be obvious to the casual observer. Service animals can do mobility, hearing, guide, medical alert/response, and other types of work to assist a person with a disability. A service animal is not a pet. Most service animals are dogs, and can be of any size or breed (or mixture of breeds). Service animals are not legally required to wear special equipment or tags. Federal law prohibits requiring proof of disability or "certification" of the service dog's training, or inquiring about the nature of the person's disability. Federal (for example, ADA 28 CFR 38.302) and state laws protect the rights of individuals with disabilities to be accompanied by their trained service animals in taxis, buses, trains, airports, airplanes, stores, restaurants, doctors' offices and hospitals, schools, courthouses, polling places, government buildings, parks, zoos, housing, and other public places.

Appendix 2
Delta Society Service
Dogs Welcome

Laws that protect the rights of people with disabilities who have trained service animals:

The federal civil rights law, the Americans With Disabilities Act (ADA), Title III, 28 CFR Sec 36, 104, defines a service animal as any animal that is individually trained to do work or perform tasks for a person with a disability (the disability might not be visible). By law, a service animal is not considered a pet. Most service animals are dogs; they can be any breed or size, and are not legally required to wear special equipment or tags. The ADA does not require proof or "certification" of the service dog's training. Service animals are trained to do specific tasks for the benefit of people with physical or mental impairments.

Federal (e.g. 28 CFR Sec 36.302) and state laws protect the rights of individuals with disabilities to be accompanied by their trained service animals in taxis, buses, trains, stores, restaurants, doctors' offices, schools, parks, hotels, and other public places. Federal laws which protect individuals with disabilities include the ADA; the Fair Housing Amendments Act (1988); Sect. 504 of the Rehabilitation Act (1973); the Air Carrier Access Act (1986); and other regulations.

State and local laws* which protect the rights of individuals who have disabilities to be accompanied by their service animals are (fill in the code numbers of the laws that apply):

*NOTE: If federal and state or local law conflict, the law that provides greater protection for the individual with the disability will prevail. For example, if state law grants access only by service dogs that do guide work, and the service dog in question performs work other than guide work, federal law will apply. The person with the disability must be permitted access with the service dog.

The person who is accompanied by the service animal is responsible for its stewardship (behavior, care, and well-being), must obey animal welfare laws (such as leash, cruelty, or other similar regulations), and is liable for any damage done by the service animal.

For more information about service animals, visit the Delta Society National Service Dog Center on Delta's Website: *www. deltasociety.org*

About the ADA, contact the U.S. Department of Justice ADA Information Line 800-514-0301 (V) 800-514-0383 (TDD)

About state and local laws, contact the State Attorney General's Office.

Service Dog Notice

Thank you for not distracting my service dog by petting or talking to him or offering him food. My well-being depends upon his ability to concentrate so that he can predict medical crises and assist me. Yes, he does get treats, playtime, lots of love, and a chance to be a "regular" dog at home, when he is off duty.

Service animals may be dogs or other animals and may be of any size, breed, or mixture of breeds. *My* service dog is a Labrador Retriever. Service animals are specially trained to assist persons with disabilities such as blindness or deafness, or with mobility issures related to disability, or medical disabilites such as epilepsy, diabetes, or psychiatric disorders. Service animals are individually trained for their specific handler and may do one or more of the following: open doors, turn on lights, predict medical crises, get help, dial a phone, pick up dropped items, help a person who has fallen get back on their feet, signal when they hear a smoke alarm or baby crying, guide a person who is blind, and much more.

Hotlines:

Learn more about service animals at the Delta Society's National Service Dog Center. (425) 226-7357 *www.deltasociety. org*. DOJ ADA Info. Line: (800) 514-0301.

Thank you to the Delta Society for granting us permission to reprint the information contained in this appendix from information obtained from their Website www.DeltaSociety.org on August 21, 2009.

Appendix 3
ADA Business BRIEF: Service Animals

In April 2002 the U.S. Department of Justice published the "ADA Business BRIEF: Service Animals." On page 162 a copy of the document is provided.

U.S. Department of Justice
Civil Rights Division
Disability Rights Section

Americans with Disabilities Act

ADA Business BRIEF:

Service Animals

Service animals are animals that are individually trained to perform tasks for people with disabilities – such as guiding people who are blind, alerting people who are deaf, pulling wheelchairs, alerting and protecting a person who is having a seizure, or performing other special tasks. Service animals are working animals, not pets.

Under the Americans with Disabilities Act (ADA), businesses and organizations that serve the public must allow people with disabilities to bring their service animals into all areas of the facility where customers are normally allowed to go. This federal law applies to <u>all</u> businesses open to the public, including restaurants, hotels, taxis and shuttles, grocery and department stores, hospitals and medical offices, theaters, health clubs, parks, and zoos.

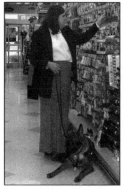

Businesses that serve the public must allow people with disabilities to enter with their service animal

■ Businesses may ask if an animal is a service animal or ask what tasks the animal has been trained to perform, but cannot require special ID cards for the animal or ask about the person's disability.

■ People with disabilities who use service animals cannot be charged extra fees, isolated from other patrons, or treated less favorably than other patrons. However, if a business such as a hotel normally charges guests for damage that they cause, a customer with a disability may be charged for damage caused by his or her service animal.

■ A person with a disability cannot be asked to remove his service animal from the premises unless: (1) the animal is out of control and the animal's owner does not take effective action to control it (for example, a dog that barks repeatedly during a movie) or (2) the animal poses a direct threat to the health or safety of others.

■ In these cases, the business should give the person with the disability the option to obtain goods and services without having the animal on the premises.

■ Businesses that sell or prepare food must allow service animals in public areas even if state or local health codes prohibit animals on the premises.

■ A business is not required to provide care or food for a service animal or provide a special location for it to relieve itself.

■ Allergies and fear of animals are generally <u>not</u> valid reasons for denying access or refusing service to people with service animals.

■ Violators of the ADA can be required to pay money damages and penalties.

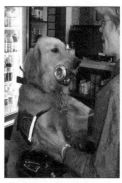

Service animals are individually trained to perform tasks for people with disabilities

If you have additional questions concerning the ADA and service animals, please call the Department's ADA Information Line at (800) 514-0301 (voice) or (800) 514-0383 (TTY) or visit the **ADA Business Connection** at **www.ada.gov**

Duplication is encouraged.   April 2002

Appendix 4
Breed Types: What's In a Name?

Different breeds and breed types possess different proportions of the five basic components that make up the compatibility profile:

- ~ Level of sociability.
- ~ Level of trainability.
- ~ Level of cooperation.
- ~ Level of activity.
- ~ Level of reactivity.

Terriers

Terriers were originally bred to be stable-dwelling dogs. Terriers were utilized as ratters and varmint chasers; they kept the barn and surrounding area free and clear of marauding bands of chicken killing, grain, stealing, and vegetable-eating animals. The terriers were not bred to be intimate companion dogs, but rather as courageous independents that went so far as to rout badgers from their dens and tangle with the likes of foxes and other larger mammals. Airedales, Scotties, Wheatens, and Yorkies are terriers.

- ~ Level of sociability: high
- ~ Level of trainability: medium–low
- ~ Level of cooperation: medium–low
- ~ Level of activity: high+
- ~ Level of reactivity: high+

Terrier behaviors with problem potential:

- ~ Very reactive; do everything with great vigor and enthusiasm. Boredom is at the root of many behavior problems.
- ~ Persistence, impatience and a strongwill.
- ~ Alertness and alarm barking abilities.
- ~ Intolerant of other animals; often chase after/fight with small animals and dogs.
- ~ Enjoy digging, chewing, ripping, and tearing.
- ~ Single-mindedness, willfully disobedience, and an uninhibited use of their mouths.

Sporting Dogs

Sporting dogs were initially bred for their ability to track, flush, and retrieve game birds. Setters, spaniels, pointers, and retrievers are sporting dogs. Cooperative by nature, they are a good choice for first time owners and families with young children.

- Level of sociability: high
- Level of trainability: high–medium
- Level of cooperation: high–medium
- Level of activity: high
- Level of reactivity: high

Sporting dog behaviors with problem potential:

- Reactive and do everything with vigor and enthusiasm. Boredom is at the root of many behavior problems.
- Roaming and wandering.
- Chasing after small animals.
- Jumping up on people and objects.

Hound Dogs

Hound dogs were initially bred for their ability to track game birds and game animals. Some hounds locate their quarry by sight; others by scent. Bloodhounds, beagles and foxhounds are scent hounds; Afghans, Scottish deerhounds, and greyhounds are sight hounds.

- ~ Level of sociability: high–medium
- ~ Level of trainability: medium–low
- ~ Level of cooperation: medium–low
- ~ Level of activity: high
- ~ Level of reactivity: high

Hound dog behaviors with problem potential:
- ~ Reactive and do everything with vigor and enthusiasm.
- ~ Independent; somewhat detached or aloof.
- ~ Whining, overbarking, or baying when excited or over-stimulated.
- ~ Roaming and wandering.
- ~ Chasing after small animals.

Working Dogs

Working dogs were initially bred to be family companions and guards; many also were utilized to pull sleds and carts. Dogs in this group tend to be large (more than 75 pounds) or giants (more than 125 pounds). They can be fiercely loyal and protective. Akitas, boxers, mastiffs, Great Danes, and mala-mutes are working dogs.
- ~ Level of sociability: medium–low
- ~ Level of trainability: medium
- ~ Level of cooperation: medium
- ~ Level of activity: medium–low
- ~ Level of reactivity: medium

Working dog behaviors with problem potential:

- ⁓ Guardians are sedentary; low level of activity.
- ⁓ Overprotective regarding possessions and/or territory.
- ⁓ Assertive, take charge nature.
- ⁓ Wary of strangers.
- ⁓ Will bite if provoked.

Herding Dogs

Herding dogs were bred for their ability to move and herd livestock through the use of predatory movements and gestures. They work closely with humans and are considered good problem-solvers and are cooperative companions. Collies, German shepherds, and corgies are herding dogs.

- ⁓ Level of sociability: high–medium
- ⁓ Level of trainability: high
- ⁓ Level of cooperation: high–medium
- ⁓ Level of activity: high
- ⁓ Level of reactivity: high

Herding dog behaviors with problem potential:

- ⁓ High energy level.
- ⁓ Barking when excited or over-stimulated.
- ⁓ Chasing after small animals.
- ⁓ Nipping at passersby and chasing after cars.

Toy Dogs

Toy dogs and companion (non-sporting) dogs were bred to be companions; they were not bred to hunt or herd or guard. They become very attached to their families. Many cannot support themselves without human intervention. Toy versions of full-size breeds retain the characteristics of the full sized counterpart. So toy poodles share the same characteristics as standard poodles; the same with toy fox terriers, etc.

- Level of sociability: high–medium
- Level of trainability: high
- Level of cooperation: high–medium
- Level of activity: high
- Level of reactivity: high

Toy dog behaviors with problem potential:

- High energy.
- Alertness and alarm barking abilities.
- Sensitive to temperature extremes.
- Dependent and demanding of attention; separation issues are not uncommon.
- Restricted diets.

Reprinted with permission:
Micky Niego/Dog's Eye View, Airmont, NY
Copyright 1991 rev. 2005

Appendix 5
Assistance Dog Tasks

By Joan Froling

Pioneers of the assistance dog concept in the 20th century have greatly enriched the lives of thousands of disabled persons worldwide with their discoveries. They devised mutually beneficial ways for assistance dogs and disabled people to work together to overcome or mitigate the difficulties imposed by certain disabling conditions.

Teamwork with a dog schooled to perform useful tasks empowers disabled individuals to function with greater self sufficiency, to prevent injuries, to summon help in a crisis, and to be aware of events in the environment. This report identifies over one hundred possible tasks that guide, hearing and service dogs can master to assist with daily life activities and safety concerns. Today, an estimated 20,000 teams in the USA and thousands in other countries from Europe to Japan to South Africa to Australia and New Zealand are reaping this legacy of empowerment.

Guide Dog Tasks

Although it is uncommon to discuss guide dog work in terms of tasks being performed, a guide dog's four to six month education involves mastering a set of tasks which, taken together, allow a blind or visually impaired individual to negotiate the unseen environment with greater safety and independence. One guide dog user of my acquaintance neatly summarized the work performed guide dogs as follows: "Guide dogs take directional commands and institute a path of travel, indicate changes in elevation, indicate and avoid oncoming traffic, navigate around obstacles and locate objects on command.

The human partner makes most of the decisions for the team, giving the dog directions and determining, after listening to the flow of traffic, the most optimal time to cross each street. Guide dogs are carefully conditioned to refuse the "Forward" command under certain circumstances where it would be unsafe to proceed, something termed "intelligent disobedience." A dog does not have the reasoning power to comprehend the inherent danger in traffic. The net effect of the conditioning, however, is a habitual reaction from the dog to specific stimuli which substantially improves team safety. It should be noted this skill deteriorates over time if the handler forgets to appropriately praise the dog for avoiding a situation. Like other assistance dogs, a guide dog relies heavily on the team leader's feedback, especially praise, to reinforce and motivate desired behaviors.

The tasks or duties listed below have been grouped into three primary skill categories. Obstacle Avoidance, Signaling Changes in Elevation and Locating Objects. The majority of guide dogs work through a harness with a U-shaped handle, that attaches to the harness and allows for vertical and some lateral movement. Some but not all may learn to do leash guiding as well. Whenever navigating around obstacles, the dog is schooled to return to the original path of travel as soon as possible. This may include moving into a road to walk around something then locating the safer pedestrian path once clear of the obstacle. Schools in North America vary in how much work is put into the tasks listed under Locating Objects. Some handlers put in extra work on "Find" command tasks with very impressive results. While a few owner trainers and private trainers include retrieving in a guide dog's repertoire, the guide dog schools no longer teach it as a mandatory skill, so it has been listed under the title, "Other Possible Tasks."

Obstacle Avoidance

- Navigate around stationary obstacles like a lamp post, parking meters, pillars.
- Navigate around hazards like an open manhole and deep potholes.
- Navigate around low hanging obstacles like awnings or a tree branch to avoid a collision.
- Avoid moving objects such as bicycles, people, strollers, shopping carts, wheelchairs.

~ Leash guiding around obstacles indoors or outdoors for a short distance.

Intelligent Disobedience as in refusing a command to go forward into the road if there is oncoming traffic or intersecting traffic in the team's path. The dog is also trained to halt, abruptly, rather than collide with a vehicle that intersects the team's path when it enters the intersection during the team's crossing.

Signal Changes in Elevation

~ Halt or Sit to indicate every curb.
~ Halt to indicate descending stairs at the top of a flight of stairs.
~ Halt to indicate steps up into a building or patio area.
~ Halt to warn of edge of subway or train platform.
~ Halt to warn of approach to edge of cliff, ditch, other outdoor drop-offs.
~ Halt when confronted by a barrier such as at construction site.
~ Intelligent disobedience—refuse a command to go forward if there is a drop-off.

Locate Objects on Command

~ Find an exit from a room; indicate door knob.
~ Find the elevator bank.
~ Find specific entrances and/or exits.
~ Find an empty seat, bench, or unoccupied area.

- Find a customary seat in a particular classroom.
- Follow a designated person such as a waiter to restaurant table, clerk to elevator, etc.
- Locate specified destination such as store in mall, hotel room or home from a distance, once all other decision points such as intersecting streets, hallways, etc. have been passed.

Other Possible Tasks

- Retrieve dropped objects.
- Find desired object like the morning newspaper on the porch.

Special Needs Guide Dog

Dogs trained solely for guide dog work are sometimes partnered with deaf blind students or mobility impaired blind students by schools specializing in such placements. In the last decade, some ground breaking experiments have taken place, combining the role of a hearing dog with that of a guide dog for deaf blind students or combining a guide dog's work with wheelchair pulling and/or other service dog tasks. This inspiring research has expanded the frontiers of knowledge as to a guide dog's capabilities and may someday give new options to disabled people with dual impairments.

Hearing Dog Tasks

Hearing dogs are schooled to alert to the specific sounds needed by their partners, primarily in the home setting. Some hearing dogs also work outside the home, alerting to specific sounds in public settings. Most are shelter dogs who receive three to six months of schooling from providers or dedicated owner trainers on sound alerts, obedience and public access manners.

It is a common misconception that hearing dogs typically alert a deaf or hard of hearing person to sounds by barking at them. Barking or growling is generally undesirable as it may not be heard by the deaf partner, will unnerve or frighten other people and if the handler shows approval, it can easily worsen the dog's fear or over protectiveness, which usually is the underlying cause of this response.

Instead of barking hearing dogs are trained to get the attention of their human partner by touch (either a nose nudge or pawing), then the dog leads the partner to the source of the specific sound. Some trainers may teach the dog to lie down next to their partner to indicate a smoke alarm after alerting the partner to the event with a touch. Leading the partner toward the sound in the case of a fire alarm may not be safe. For that reason a number of handlers prefer to have the dog indicate the smoke alarm indirectly and to wait for the human to decide what the next response should be. Responding to specific sounds in public or in a moving vehicle also requires a slight adjustment of the customary response to suit the location.

Some hearing dogs master additional tasks, enhancing communication between family members. This can be especially helpful in households with a child, those where more than one member has a hearing impairment or households where one or more members are non verbal.

Alert to Specific Sounds at Home

- Doorbell ringing.
- Knock on front door.
- Rapping on patio door or window.
- Smoke alarm sounding.
- Wind up minute timer, oven or microwave timer going off.
- Baby crying.
- Family member or other calling the name of the dog's partner.
- Child calling "mommy" (or other name, if applicable, such as daddy, grandpa, aunt).
- Phone ringing.
- Alarm clock buzzing.
- Computer equipment beeps.
- Horn honking in garage or driveway.
- Arrival of school bus.

Alert to Specific Sounds Away From Home

- Siren of police car, fire truck or ambulance and indicate direction.

- ~ Smoke alarm in workplace.
- ~ Distinguish phone ringing on partner's desk at work from all other phones in workplace.
- ~ Name of partner if coworker, friend, family member calls out that name.
- ~ Cell phone or beeper.
- ~ Smoke alarm in hotel or work.
- ~ Fire drill at school or work.
- ~ Vehicle honking to attract attention.

Other Possible Tasks

- ~ Retrieve unheard dropped objects like keys, coins, or other objects.
- ~ To enhance security when the team arrives home after dark, the dog enters the home first to turn on a light, nudging the metal base of a lamp with a touch lamp device.
- ~ Carry a note from the partner to another household member, searching the house to find that individual.
- ~ Carry messages between spouses, utilizing objects which signify dinner is ready or that the person needs help right away, and so forth.
- ~ Have the dog find and return with the hearing impaired person.
- ~ Warn of a vehicle approaching from behind, or making a sudden turn. A task that applies the intelligent disobedience principle to hearing dog work.

Service Dog Tasks

Service dogs generally receive six months to a year of schooling on tasks, obedience and public access manners. Most dogs placed by non profits since the 1970's have been trained to assist people who have a wide variety of mobility impairments. Some teams have mastered up to fifty tasks, enjoying the challenge of such an advanced education. The list of tasks in this section are a broad sampling of what has been developed over the past quarter century to address daily living needs and safety issues.

A number of the traditional tasks listed below are proving useful to individuals with hidden disabilities such as a seizure disorder, a psychiatric disorder, a potentially life threatening medical problem or conditions which cause chronic pain. Creative providers, graduates and owner trainers who are expanding the service dog concept into these additional areas will hopefully share the experimental tasks they develop with the larger community someday, providing task training particulars so others can benefit. In some cases, a responsible third party, usually a parent or a spouse, facilitates the interactions between a disabled person and his or her service dog to optimize the benefits to be obtained from including a service dog in the independent living plan of that individual.

For specific tasks to address specific symptoms of disabilities like Parkinson's Disease or MS or Epilepsy or any other disabling condition, one option is to research the subject by consulting with training providers familiar with those conditions. A second option is to send out a specific information request on email lists in the assistance dog field, gathering a variety of input. As a precaution, a second query, asking trainers and handlers for recommended ethical and /or safety guidelines in connection with any task being considered, may yield valuable input to assist with assessing the appropriateness of the suggested task for a particular team. A third option is to search archives for newspaper stories, magazine articles, television newscasts and documentaries which may focus on a particular disability or provider or type of assistance dog. Books on training guide, hearing or service dogs, autobiographies, biographies and works of fiction may in some cases, provide additional information on the desired topic.

A myth that ought to be challenged is the belief on the part of some that service dogs are only for the most severely impaired or end stage of a degenerative disease like MS. Someone who is considered much more moderately disabled, struggling with the difficulties of living alone, maintaining a job or raising a family could find teamwork with a highly trained service dog to be of enormous benefit in achieving the goal of remaining as self sufficient as possible. A number of tasks enumerated in this section could empower such individuals to conserve energy, reduce or avoid pain, minimize dependency on loved ones, prevent injuries or get help in a crisis.

Retrieve Based Tasks

- Bring portable phone to any room in house.
- Bring in groceries—up to ten canvas bags.
- Unload suitable grocery items from canvas sacks.
- Fetch a beverage from a refrigerator or cupboard.
- Fetch food bowl(s).

- Pick up dropped items such as coins, keys etc., in any location.
- Bring clothes, shoes, or slippers laid out to assist with dressing.
- Unload towels, other items from dryer.
- Retrieve purse from hall, desk, dresser or back of van.
- Assist to tidy house or yard—pickup, carry, deposit designated items.
- Fetch basket with medication and/or beverage from cupboard.
- Seek and find teamwork—direct the dog with hand signals, vocal cues to: retrieve an unfamiliar object out of partner's reach, locate TV remote control, select one of several VCR tapes atop TV cabinet, other surfaces.
- Remove VCR tape from machine after eject button pushed.
- Use target stick to retrieve an indicated item off shelves in stores retrieve one pair of shoes from a dozen in closet.
- Use laser pointer to target an item to be retrieved.
- Drag Cane from its customary location to another room.
- Pick up and return cane if falls off back of wheelchair.
- Pickup or fetch Canadian crutches from customary location.
- Drag walker back to partner.
- Fetch wheelchair when out of reach.

Carrying Based Tasks (Non Retrieval)

- ~ Move bucket from one location to another, indoors & outdoors.
- ~ Lug a basket of items around the house.
- ~ Transport items downstairs or upstairs to a specific location.
- ~ Carry item(s) from the partner to a care-giver or family member in another room.
- ~ Send the dog to obtain food or other item from a care-giver and return with it.
- ~ Dog carries a prearranged object to care-giver as a signal help is needed.
- ~ Carry items following a partner using a walker, other mobility aids.
- ~ Pay for purchases at high counters.
- ~ Transfer merchandise in bag from a clerk to a wheelchair user's lap.
- ~ Carry mail or newspaper into the house.

Deposit Based Tasks

- ~ Put trash, junk mail into a wastebasket or garbage can.
- ~ Deposit empty soda pop can or plastic bottle into recycling bin.
- ~ Assist partner to load clothing into top loading washing machine.
- ~ Dirty food bowl [dog's] put into kitchen sink.
- ~ Put silverware, non breakable dishes, plastic glasses in sink.

- Deliver items to "closet" (use a floor marker to indicate drop location).
- Deposit dog toys into designated container.
- Put prescription bag, mail, other items on counter top.

Tug Based Tasks

- Open cupboard doors with attached strap.
- Open drawers via strap.
- Open refrigerator door with a strap or suction cup device.
- Open interior doors via a strap with device to turn knob.
- Answer doorbell and open front door with strap attached to lever handle.
- Open or close sliding glass door with a strap or other tug devices.
- Shut restroom door that opens outward via a leash tied to doorknob.
- Close stall door that opens outward in restroom by delivering end of the leash to partner.
- Shut interior home, office doors that open outward.
- Shut motel room exterior door that opens inward.
- Assist to remove shoes, slippers, sandals.
- Tug socks off without biting down on foot.
- Remove slacks, sweater, coat.
- Drag heavy coat, other items to closet.
- Drag laundry basket through house with a strap.
- Drag bedding to the washing machine.
- Wrestle duffle bag or other objects from the van into the house.

- Pull a drapery cord to open or close drapes.
- Assist to close motel room drapes by tugging on edge near bottom of drape, backing up.
- Operate rope device that lifts blanket and sheet or recovers disabled person when he or she becomes too hot or cold.
- Alternatively, take edge of a blanket and move backwards, tugging to remove it or assist someone to pull the blanket up to their chin if cold.

Nose Nudge Based Tasks

- Cupboard door or drawers—nudge shut.
- Dryer door—hard nudge.
- Stove drawer—push it shut.
- Dishwasher door—put muzzle under open door, flip to shut.
- Refrigerator and freezer door—close with nudge.
- Call 911 on K-9 rescue phone—push the button.
- Operate button or push plate on electric commercial doors.
- Turn on light switches.
- Push floor pedal device to turn on lamp.
- Turn on metal based lamps with touch-lamp device installed—nudge base.
- Assist wheelchair user to regain sitting position if slumped over.
- Help put paralyzed arm back onto the armrest of wheelchair.

- Return paralyzed foot to the foot board of a wheelchair if it is dislodged.

Pawing Based Tasks (Some Dogs Prefer It to Nose Nudge)

- Cupboard door—shut it with one paw.
- Dryer door—shut it with one paw.
- Refrigerator and freezer door—one forepaw or both.
- Call 911 on K-9 rescue phone—hit button with one paw.
- Operate light switch on wall—jump up, paw the switch
- Depress floor pedal device to turn on appliance(s) or lamp.
- Jump up to paw elevator button (steady dog if he tries it on slippery tile floor).
- Operate push plate on electric commercial doors.
- Close heavy front door, other doors—jump up, use both forepaws.

Bracing Based Tasks (No Harness)

- Transfer assistance from wheelchair to bed, toilet, bathtub or van seat—hold Stand Stay position, then brace on command, enabling partner to keep their balance during transfer.
- Assist to walk step by step, brace between each step, from wheelchair to nearby seat.

- Position self and brace to help partner catch balance after partner rises from a couch or other seats in a home or public setting.
- Prevent fall by bracing on command if the partner needs help recovering balance.
- Steady partner getting in or out of the bathtub.
- Assist partner to turn over in bed; have appropriate backup plan.
- Pull up partner with a strap [tug of war style] from floor to feet on command, then brace till partner catches balance.

Harness Based Tasks, Mobility Assistance

Only appropriate for large sturdy adult dogs with sound joints, proper training.

- Assist moving wheelchair on flat [partner holds onto harness pull strap] avoiding obstacles.
- Work cooperatively with partner to get the wheelchair up a curb cut or mild incline; handler does as much of the work as possible, never asking the dog to attempt an incline unaided.
- Haul open heavy door, holding it ajar using six foot lead attached to back of harness, other end of lead attached to door handle or to a suction cup device on a glass door.
- Tow ambulatory partner up inclines [harness with rigid handle or pull strap may be used].
- Brace on command to prevent ambulatory partner from stumbling (rigid handle).

~ Help ambulatory partner to climb stairs, pulling then bracing on each step (rigid handle or harness with pull strap may be used to assist partner to mount a step or catch balance).

~ Pull partner out of aisle seat on plane, then brace until partner catches balance (harness with a rigid handle and a pull strap, or pull strap only).

~ Brace, counter balance work too, assisting ambulatory partner to walk; the partner pushes down on the rigid handle as if it were a cane, after giving warning command, when needed.

~ Help ambulatory partner to walk short distance, brace between each step (rigid handle).

~ Transport textbooks, business supplies or other items up to 50 lbs. in a wagon or collapsible cart, weight limit depends on dog's size, physical fitness, type of cart, kind of terrain.

~ Backpacking—customary weight limit is 15% of the dog's total body weight; 10% if a dog performing another task, such as wheelchair pulling in addition to backpacking; total weight includes harness (average 3–4 lbs.). Load must be evenly distributed to prevent chafing.

Other Kinds of Assistance in Crisis

~ Bark for help on command.

~ Find the care-giver on command, lead back to location of disabled partner.

- Put forepaws in lap of wheelchair user, hold that upright position so wheelchair user can access medication or cell phone or other items in the backpack.
- Wake up partner if smoke alarm goes off, assist to nearest exit.

Medical Assistant Tasks (Sample)

- Operate push button device to call 911, an ambulance service or another person to help in a crisis; let emergency personnel into home and lead to partner's location
- Fetch insulin kit, respiratory assist device or medication from customary place during a medical crisis.
- Lie down on partner's chest to produce a cough, enabling patient to breath, when suction machine and/or care-giver unavailable.

Comments? Questions? Contact Joan: iaadp@aol.com
Copyrighted April 16, 2001
Contact author for reprint permission. *www.iaadp.org*
May not be published or reproduced in part or in its entirety without reprint permission.

With permission to reprint granted by Joan Froling, September 3, 2009.

Appendix 6
Service Dog Tasks for Psychiatric Disabilities

Tasks to mitigate certain disabling illnesses classified as mental impairments under the Americans With Disabilities Act. Author: Joan Froling, Trainer Consultant—Sterling Service Dogs.

Service Dog Tasks for Panic Disorder, PTSD, and Depression

According to the Americans With Disabilities Act (ADA), a service animal must be individually trained to do work or perform tasks of benefit to a disabled individual in order to be legally elevated from pet status to service animal status. It is the specially trained tasks or work performed on command or cue that legally exempts a service dog [service animal] and his disabled handler from the "No Pets Allowed" policies of stores, restaurants and other places of public accommodation under the ADA.

The following list identifies a number of tasks a service dog could be trained to do that would serve to mitigate the effects of a disabling condition classified as a psychiatric disability. In particular, the tasks were developed for those who become disabled by Panic Disorder, Post Traumatic Stress Disorder (PTSD), or Depression, conditions attributed to a brain chemistry malfunction. The List also contains some activities that may be useful as a coping mechanism, but would not stand up in a court of law as "a trained task that mitigates the effect of a disability," and those will be marked with a Disclaimer to provide guidance to a therapist and patient on that issue. The author, a mobility impaired service dog trainer who has been deeply involved in the assistance dog field for many years, initiated research into this new kind of assistance dog in 1997. She became familiar with these disorders through the input of early pioneers of the psychiatric service dog concept. Subsequent research has involved garnering input from experts in psychology and psychiatry and from patients to gain a better understanding of the symptoms, treatment goals, and ways in which partnership with a service dog might become a valuable adjunct to conventional therapy.

In addition to task training, it should also be recognized that housebreaking, basic obedience training and mastering the behaviors of no nuisance barking, no aggressive behavior, and no inappropriate sniffing or intrusion into another person or dog's space are an essential part of educating any dog for a career as a service dog.

Clarification: While a dog's companionship may offer emotional support, comfort or a sense of security, this in and of itself does NOT qualify as a "trained task" or "work" under the ADA, thus it does not give a disabled person the legal right to take that dog out in public as a legitimate service dog. Setting up a realistic training plan to transform a dog with a suitable temperament into an obedient, task trained service dog is the only way to legally qualify a dog to become a service dog [service animal] whose disabled handler is legally permitted to take the dog into restaurants, grocery stores, hospitals, medical offices and other places of public accommodation. I recommend reading IAADP's Minimum Training Standards for Public Access for further guidance at *www.iaadp.org.*

Gender: While I refer to a dog as "him" in this article rather than using the word "it," both genders can be equally good at a service dog career if the dog has the temperament to calmly tolerate loud noises, other animals, strangers reaching out to pet the dog without permission and the other challenges of working with a service dog out in public.

Assistance Work or Tasks for Psychiatric Disabilities

I. Assistance in a Medical Crisis
II. Treatment Related Assistance
III. Assistance Coping With Emotional Overload
IV. Security Enhancement Tasks

I. Assistance in a Medical Crisis

A service dog can learn a number of helpful tasks to assist his partner to cope during a sudden flare up of symptoms, medication side effects, or in a situation requiring outside help.

Bring Medication to Alleviate Symptoms

- ~ Dog assists partner to cope with nausea, cramps, dizziness, other medication side effects or the fear paralysis of PTSD or the sudden waves of terror, chest pains and respiratory distress of a severe panic attack by fetching antidote medication to alleviate the severity of the symptoms.
- ~ Dog is trained to retrieve a small canvas bag with medication from a specific location that he is schooled to go to on command, such as a closet floor, bathroom vanity or shelf.
- ~ Dog can be trained to go tug open a cupboard door and retrieve a basket or satchel with medication if access to the first location is blocked by the door to the room being shut
- ~ Dog can be trained to locate a purse with medication in home, office or on a hotel room dresser, desk or chair by following directional commands, then drag-deliver it to partner.

Bring a Beverage so Human Partner Can Swallow Medication

This complex task involves a sequence of skills, takes four to six months to master.

Dog can be trained to fetch a beverage to enable the human partner to swallow the medication.

Must master the skills of: 1) going to the kitchen from another room to pull open a refrigerator door or cupboard door with a strap, 2) picking up the beverage from refrigerator shelf before the door swings shut, 3) carrying cold beverage to the partner in another room, 4) going back, if need be, to shut the refrigerator door or instead: 5) fetch a basket or some other container from a kitchen cupboard with a beverage and other items; may also contain antidote type medication in a vial with a childproof cap.

Bring the Emergency Phone During a Crisis

Enables the human partner to contact a doctor, therapist or others in a support system when experiencing alarming medication side effects, terror or respiratory distress from a panic attack, or a flashback. An individual suffering from depression, possibly with suicidal ideation, also needs to be able to reach a supporting person or agency. Retrieval of the portable phone can be very useful in other situations too. (Training Note: this should be made a "place command," as asking a dog to visually search the house is unreliable, especially if the phone is left on a counter or piece of furniture above the dog's line of sight. It is best to locate the charger unit on the floor in a room with two entrances. If possible, the emergency phone should never be used except during practice sessions. This will ensure its availability during a crisis.)

Dog is trained to bring the handler a portable phone. If the room where the emergency phone is permanently located has two entrances, the dog should also be specifically taught to find the second entrance in case the first is blocked. The end goal is to train a service dog to bring the phone to any room in the house when needed on command.

Answer the Doorbell

When situations occur in which the handler urgently needs help but cannot get to the front door to let someone into the home due to physical incapacity from drug interactions, injuries that occurred due to lightheadedness, fainting, other side effects, or illness, the service dog could assist by opening the front door and escorting emergency personnel or a member of the support system to the handler's location.

Dog is trained to tug strap on a lever handle to open the front door to let in emergency personnel or members of support system on command or in response to the doorbell itself. The dog is trained to escort the person to the handler's location.

Call 911 or Suicide Hotline on K-9 Rescue Phone

People with physical disabilities have reported going through periods of severe depression and not a few admit they've contemplated suicide. Those with a mental disability like PTSD are equally susceptible to developing this mood disorder or experiencing a sudden exacerbation of its symptoms. Scientists view it as a biological problem, not purely psychological. With some persons, the condition becomes a lifelong struggle. A service dog can improve the safety of his partner whenever the mood disorder becomes life threatening. One task to consider is schooling the dog to operate the K-9 Rescue phone to summon help during a crisis. (Available at *www.ablephone.com*.)

The dog is trained to call 911/any preprogrammed number by depressing the huge white button on a K-9 Rescue speakerphone with his paw.

Bring Help Indoors and Provide Speech Impairment Assistance

Symptoms of extreme terror, shortness of breath or the wrong dosage of a major tranquilizer like thorazine are a few of the reasons why the patient may need to summon help and may not be able to give a verbal command. Suggested tasks can be taught with hand signals so as to enable the team to communicate in such a crisis. These tasks may be useful at other times too.

- Dog taught to bark at a speaker-phone on a hand signal. (As pre-planned with the patient's family, therapist or other members of his or her Support System.)
- Dog is trained to go nudge a certain household member on command in a crisis.
- Dog taught to carry a note to a spouse or another household member on command.
- Dog should learn to open interior doors with a lever handle and strap, or knob-to-lever conversion device so he could exit bedroom or office to carry out a "get help" task.

Summon Help from a Secretary, Coworker, or Supervisor

- Dog can learn to carry a message to designated support person or relief person in an office or retail setting. Could also learn to bark to summon designated employee as prearranged.

There are a variety of ways a dog could summon help in the workplace. It will depend on the situation and/or particular tasks he has been schooled to perform.

Provide Balance Assistance on Stairs

Goal is to prevent a serious injury from a fall. Very useful if the person experiences dizziness due to medication side effects of psychotropic drugs. Task also can assist individuals who experience dizziness or weakness due to not eating because of major depression. Rest one hand on the withers of a large sturdy dog to steady oneself on each step, harness optional.

Large dog is trained to assist his partner to climb or descend stairs with greater safety, by halting on each step, then bracing himself on command to steady the person when the person takes their next step. Dog must learn to only take one step, not 2 or 3 at a time.

Assist Person to Rise and Steady That Person

When the partner must cope with weakness or medication side effects like dizziness, a service dog schooled in balance support work can prevent a fall or assist the partner to get up after a fall occurs. (Training Note: Introduce one's weight gradually to a beginner; only reward correct responses. One hand should be on the dog's withers, the other may lightly rest on his rump. Push down ONLY on withers so human's weight borne by the dog's powerful shoulders in the few seconds it takes to boost oneself to a standing position. Ethically, the service dog must be an appropriate size for this work—e.g. 55 lbs. or more)

Dog assists someone to get up from the floor or a chair by holding a Stand Stay position and stiffening his muscles on command, bracing himself to offer counter resistance for balance support when the partner places one hand on the dog's withers and gets up.

Dog is further trained to Brace on command, stiffening body, acts as the Rock of Gibraltar, for at least ten seconds, to steady someone as soon as they rise to their feet instead of darting away or sitting, so as to prevent an accidental loss of balance.

Balance Support to Ambulatory Partner

Balance support skills in a dog of suitable size can be a valuable asset when medication side effects or symptoms suddenly put the individual at risk of falling. These tasks can be performed off leash, without a harness, indoors. Frequent practice needed to keep these skills viable.

A large dog can be schooled to prevent a fall by stiffening his body to provide counter balance help if a person suddenly stumbles or feels dizzy. Ethically, you must give a warning with a command like "Brace" before putting weight on the dog's withers, so he can stiffen his muscles first.

Large dogs can be trained to assist a person to ambulate to the nearest seat, step by step, bracing after each step to allow the person to steady oneself when taking next step.

Respond to Smoke Alarm if Partner Unresponsive

Someone who has disassociation episodes with PTSD might be an excellent candidate for the same kind of training given to a dog who must alert a heavily sedated partner (as described in next section) whenever a smoke alarm goes off. If he or she has disassociated and there's a fire, the dog can learn to respond to the sound by nudging the partner persistently till handler is aware enough to reward the dog and dial 911. However, if the person typically is not responsive to nudges while in such a state, the trainer could teach the dog to go to a K-9 Rescue Phone [see *www.ablephone.com*] and paw the button to dial 911 in response to a smoke alarm's sound. Local 911 computer can be programmed, if handler requests it, to instruct operator that if no voice is heard, to assume the service dog in residence is placing the call due to a life threatening emergency. If the human partner happens to be fully aware when the smoke alarm goes off, he or she can easily intervene to disconnect the call after praising the dog for responding appropriately to that particular sound. Will need once a month practice sessions to maintain this skill in a service dog. (Training Note: may program this phone to call your own number so 911 isn't bothered during practice sessions.)

- Dog is trained to persistently nudge partner to alert to smoke alarm whenever needed.
- Alternately, the dog is trained to call 911 on K9 Rescue phone if smoke alarm goes off.

Backpacking Medical Supplies / Information

Some may protest that this should not be counted as a task and I agree. It deserves a mention, though, because it is so useful to assistance dog partners who may be in need of the items being carried by the service dog. While most dogs will calmly permit strangers such as emergency personnel to search the backpacks in a medical crisis so they can obtain the human partner's Medic Alert information, (if any) or the dog's Emergency care-giver Information card or other instructions the dog may be carrying in case the need arises, some dogs will require one or more desensitization sessions to socialize them till they will tolerate a stranger searching the packs.

Dog carries Medication in the backpack in case of a panic attack, other symptoms. Also may carry a Beverage, plus a Cell Phone or Beeper, and Instructions For Emergency Personnel, such as Who To Call if a patient is having a PTSD disassociation episode, a flashback, or if serious medication side effects, an injury or other problems should deprive the handler of the ability to provide important information about the team. DISCLAIMER: Please understand Backpacking is NOT a task that will legally "count" as a trained task acceptable in a court of law as proof the dog meets the legal definition of a service animal under the Americans With Disabilities Act (ADA). It is simply an optional extra, a "bonus aid," which any dog lover, disabled or non disabled, may enjoy. Such items could be carried in a purse or fanny pack, so it is a matter of personal choice.

II. Treatment Related Assistance

Tasks in this section suggest additional ways in which a service dog might assist a patient to cope with aspects of living with a psychiatric disability. This may include tasks to help a partner mitigate chronic or intermittent medication side effects or to take his or her medication on schedule or to assist with symptoms experienced in spite of the treatment being received.

Medication Reminder at Certain Time of Day

Success has been reported in making use of a dog's internal alarm clock, to remind the partner to take medication on time. Teach the dog to expect to be fed or to have a cookie break or to go for a walk at the same time every day. Some service dogs will pick up their food bowl or leash and bring it to the partner at the same time each day, as if they can read the clock. Other dogs may nudge or bark at the partner, begging for their dinner, treat or walk at the expected time. Submissive dogs should be encouraged to "bother" the partner with nudging or pawing at that time of day. If always rewarded, this behavior becomes habitual, a task that serves to remind the partner that it is time to stop an ongoing activity and to take the prescribed medication.

Dog trained to interrupt the partner at a certain time of day or night. Dog encouraged by training to "nag" a person till he receives the anticipated food or cookie or walk. This increases the probability the partner will get up to take the pill when it is due. Can be a task in the home and perhaps in the workplace or at school if circumstances permit.

Speech Impairment Task Away From Home

If a loss of speech may occur due to side effects of a major tranquilizer or anti-depressant medication or PTSD or a panic attack, consider carrying a card that explains what is happening to you, to show to a security guard, teacher, employer or bus driver as needed. This card can reassure them you do NOT need help or, conversely, ask them to call somebody on your behalf. It can be a postcard size or business card size, laminated. Also it is useful to have a similar card to explain your dog is a service dog and your civil rights whenever you are unable to do so.

- Dog is trained to deliver a laminated card to someone his partner points to.

Coping With the Medication Side Effect— Dry Mouth Woes

Some medications cause side effects that are more than a minor nuisance. For example, with the condition of dry-mouth the patient's speech will become progressively impaired if the person does not have a beverage constantly available as an antidote. It is highly useful to have a dog trained to fetch a beverage from a kitchen cupboard or refrigerator, so the person does not have to interrupt an important activity to get a refill to rehydrate one's self.

- ⁓ Dog is trained to retrieve a beverage from a Cupboard or Refrigerator by hand signal.

Alert Sedated Partner to the Cry of Someone in Distress

Some psychotropic medication cause deep sedation, during which it is almost impossible to regain consciousness. Other medications for pain, seizures or anxiety also can cause sedative side effects. If a parent or care-giver who takes such medication has a service dog trained to perform this outstanding "get help" task, the child or a spouse or an elderly parent who calls out in the middle of the night for the dog's partner won't be calling out in vain.

Similar to a hearing dog responding to an alarm clock; dog jumps on bed, persistently licks face or nudges partner till the partner wakes up, gives the dog a reward.

The dog leads the groggy adult to whomever is calling for the dog's human partner.

Wake Sedated Partner, Alerting to Doorbell

Waiting for a plumber, other repairmen, a delivery truck which may or may not show up can be problematic. One cannot skip a dose or forego medication if panic attack symptoms begin. Schooling a dog to wake up his partner in response to doorbell chimes can solve the dilemma.

Similar to hearing dog alert. Dog trained to awaken sleeping partner who takes medication with sedative side effects and lead that person to the source of the sound.

Alert Sedated Partner to Smoke Alarm and Assist to Exit

The dog can be trained to persist in arousing a person if sedative side effect prevents person from responding appropriately to the smoke alarm in an emergency. The dog can show the way to nearest exit, tug the door strap on a lever handle to open the door, not because a dog understands "danger" but due to many practice sessions that condition the service dog to perform this habitual sequence of tasks whenever the dog hears a smoke alarm going off.

- Dog is trained to alert the human partner and to persist with the method taught such as face licking or nuzzling till the person sits up, rewards dog, indicating awake state.
- Dog is trained to lead his partner to the front door (or some other pre-selected exit)
- Dog opens exit door with a pull strap in case the partner is too sedated to think clearly.

Harness Work With Ambulatory Partner

In spite of treatment, some people experience such a degree of fear or panic they report they frequently stumble as they cannot pay attention to their footing at such times. Others report chronic or intermittent dizziness that results in falls unless they can hang onto a family member's arm, a dependency that can restrict access to the outside world to only a few hours a week. Veterans with PTSD may experience balance problems from another issue, such as a traumatic brain injury, vertigo etc., as do civilians with psychiatric disorders according to programs working with such individuals. Use of a balance support harness with a rigid handle custom sized to bridge the distance between the withers of a large sturdy dog and the partner's height can be a solution that reduces the risk of injurious falls. In addition to the counter balance skill, such dogs could be trained like a guide dog to halt at curbs, steps, etc. to signal a risky elevation change to assist inattentive handlers to avoid a fall. The handle itself also enhances the partner's sense of "connectedness" with the service dog, which for some is a highly rated side benefit according to anecdotal input. Not everyone with a psychiatric disability needs or wants this optional task, but I mention it as it has been beneficial in some cases.

Ethical programs/trainers/handlers only select large dogs, 55–150 lbs., matched to the partner's height, weight, for this work. Physical soundness is essential, to prevent any harm to the dog from doing it. Dogs who must cope with the weight of partner, bracing on a frequent basis on outings, are customarily required to pass an orthopedic exam with x-rays for hip and elbow dysplasia to rule out these crippling joint diseases prior to counter balance training. A proper fitting harness with padding on pressure points [see *www.circle-e.net* for an example], is also essential. Such harnesses run from an estimated $70 for pre-made gear up to $500 for custom sizing and amenities like a lightweight airline metal handle, fold down option, ergonomic styled grip and a pressure relief saddle.

NOTE: The use of smaller dogs (10 lbs–50 lbs) for balance support by having the dog drag the owner along, keeping the leash taut, results in the owner putting a heavy strain on the poor dog's neck through the collar. Whether or not it aids the owner to keep his or her balance is irrelevant, for it is ethically viewed as abusive treatment of an assistance dog, which is inexcusable.

Large, physically sound dogs can be trained to assist a partner who would benefit from such aid to reduce the risk of falls while walking. It is customary to use a harness with a rigid handle designed to ergonomically distribute the weight of the partner, whenever the partner pushes down on the handle, after giving a "Brace" command to signal the dog to go into action and provide counter balance help.

III. Coping With Emotional Overload

This section details specific work or tasks a service dog can be trained to perform to assist the handler with emotionally disabling symptoms other than a fear of a violent crime reoccurring. It suggests strategies to use at home or in the workplace or in public to cope with and recover from an emotional overload. It also looks at ways to prevent feelings of panic from escalating. Quite frankly, most dogs do not rush sympathetically to the side of a human to comfort the person when he or she becomes tearful or trembles with fear or experiences a panic attack. The calm detachment of many dogs enables them to learn and carry out tasks to earn a reward. Dogs who initially show avoidance behavior can often be desensitized to emotional reactions if highly food motivated and then learn a task. Such tasks if practiced on a regular basis will empower the disabled individual to do something constructive about very unwelcome or inappropriate emotional reactions rather than feeling helpless and overwhelmed when they occur.

Provide Tactile Stimulation to Disrupt the Overload

Tasks that can provide a tactile distraction from a disorder's symptoms have proven to be quite useful in emotional overload situations. One or more of the tasks listed below may put a stop to unwelcome reactions in the workplace, classroom or out in public. In addition, for those experiencing nightmares, night terrors, hypnagogic hallucinations or flashbacks, tactile stimulation can provide a vitally important reality affirmation when the partner summons the dog. While some dogs may naturally perform a behavior, it takes schooling to transform it into a task the dog will do immediately on command, reliable even in the presence of distractions, at any location where needed.

Dog is trained to vigorously lick someone's face on command to bring his partner to full awareness, just as seizure response dogs can be trained to do when their partner is extremely groggy after a grand mal, which shortens the recovery time. This unpleasant tactile stimulation also can divert the partner's attention from something that triggers tears or other inappropriate emotional reactions in school or a workplace.

Dogs can be trained to get up from under a desk or behind chair on command or a cue like patting one's knee to use nose to nudge the partner which disrupts sudden overload. To assist the person to regain composure, the dog must learn to be obnoxiously persistent with the nudging till the partner recovers enough to respond with the desired reward.

A caregiver can adapt this nudging task into a "Go See (David)" command so the service dog will go over and perform this nudging to interrupt inappropriate repetitive behavior that a child on the autism spectrum may engage in. If a dog is large and persistent, unfazed by emotional outbursts, this nudging could also disrupt a child's tantrum or assist someone crying or having a flashback to recover faster.

Dog is asked to get up on the bed and to tolerate a hug or to snuggle next to the person to permit the person to pet the dog till the person feels better. DISCLAIMER: Please understand this last activity is NOT going to legally "count" as a trained task acceptable in a court of law as proof the dog meets the legal definition of a service animal. It is something that may not require any training for an affectionate pet. These are interactions of the sort any dog lover, disabled or non disabled, may find beneficial when emotionally upset. Such comfort is considered to be a "bonus" by service dog handlers. Since some individuals prefer this interaction to a "snap them out of it" task, it seems worth mentioning this is an option.

Break the Spell and/or Combat Sedative Side Effects

If tasks which provide tactile stimulation don't suffice, this "break the spell" strategy frequently helps in certain situations. After experiencing night terrors, repeated nightmares, hypnagogic hallucinations, sickening memories or suicidal thoughts that can't be shaken, an abrupt change of scene to break the spell can be the best medicine. By going into another room with your service dog, asking him to perform tasks, it will make it possible to get one's mind off what has just occurred, or in the case of intrusive thoughts due to PTSD or suicidal ideation, to disrupt what is still occurring. It can also help a person to shake off the grogginess of sedative side effects.

- Dog is trained to turn on bedroom or hall light or other lights, if needed.
- Dog is trained to bring the TV Remote on command, which enables the partner to switch on the set, utilizing the startle effect of this sudden audio and visual stimuli plus this additional teamwork to vanquish extremely distressing thoughts, feelings and images. It can prevent a relapse of sleep disturbances.
- Dog is trained to fetch a Beverage and/or Medication, becoming the focal point of his partner's attention as he carries out the command(s). The concentration required for a successful delivery and the heartwarming cooperation of one's service dog can disrupt the deeply disturbing thoughts that have taken hold of the partner's mind. It strengthens the partner's ability to remain in the "here and now."

~ Dog or partner initiates a game of fetch or tug with a toy, which assists the person to resist sedative side effects and may break the grip of obsessive thoughts or memories.

DISCLAIMER: this kind of play will not count as a "trained task" in a court of law and it does NOT legally transform a pet into a service animal, as untrained dogs can do it. It could serve as an alternative coping strategy if a dog lacks the schooling to perform the suggested tasks.

Wake Up Human Partner for Work or School

Panic Disorder, PTSD, Major Depression can disrupt normal thought processes. The person may not want to get up for work or school, as it means he or she will be returning to a place that he or she blames as being responsible for the panic attack or flashback. Depression can cause apathy or a desire to withdraw rather than face the world. Success has been noted in fighting back against avoidance behavior, apathy or withdrawal by having the service dog respond like a hearing dog to the alarm clock in the morning. It may also be possible to train the dog to go by his internal alarm clock to eagerly awaken the person at a certain hour of the day, through use of a feeding schedule or if not motivated by food, by the promise of a walk. After sitting up to reward the dog for performing this task, the sight of the dog's happy face, the extra tactile stimulation as he eagerly anticipates a walk or play session or a bowl of dog food can motivate a dog lover to fight back against avoidance behavior or apathy and get out of bed, which is why having a dog perform this task is arguably superior to just using an easily silenced alarm clock.

- Dog responds to alarm clock like a hearing dog. Wakes up his partner by getting up on the bed, then nuzzling the partner with a cold nose or by licking the partner's face.
- Dog can be trained to wake a person up according to "internal alarm clock," at same time every day.

Prevent or Combat Emotional Overload in Workplace

These tasks may have an incidental therapeutic benefit, giving a feeling of solace to some handlers, but their primary purpose is to empower the human partner to recover and sustain emotional control in settings where uncontrolled emotional reactions are unacceptable. Use licking or nose nudging task as described in earlier Tactile Stimulation section.

During a business meeting, a dog can assist his partner by unobtrusively maintaining a Sit Stay without sliding into the Down position, out of reach. A toy breed could be told to perform a Down Stay in the partner's lap. The human partner utilizes a relaxation technique such as giving the dog a massage or simply strokes the dog's fur to calm self, so he or she can to continue to take part in the meeting. DISCLAIMER: Please understand that obedience to a Stay command to allow petting or the voluntary presence of a dog for petting is NOT a service dog task that will legally count as a trained task in a court of law. Nevertheless, I mention it here as a "Bonus Aid," as it provides an emotional benefit that anecdotal reports suggest can be valuable to someone experiencing a panic attack, an anxiety attack or other kinds of emotional upsets.

Providing an Excuse to Leave Upsetting Situation

The following task may be an effective coping mechanism in the workplace and elsewhere, preventing a loss of self control in front of others. The dog is trained to assist the person to escape from a certain conversation, a room, or a building to earn a reward. In response to a surreptitious hand signal or another cue, the dog performs an attention seeking behavior such as nuzzling and licking the partner's hand or jumping up to disrupt a query or confrontation that triggers an emotional overload. This provides the human partner with a plausible reason for taking a break from an intolerable situation with a boss, client or co-worker, thus saving face or the job. Some breeds can learn to vocalize on command, whining or "talking" or giving a short yip in response to a surreptitious hand signal, (for example, flexing the first digit of the forefinger on your right hand). This increases the impression that it is urgent for the disabled person to take dog outside before the dog has an accident in the office due to the dog's alleged stomach or bowel upset.

- Dog trained to "bother" his partner with pawing or a nose nudge, or by jumping up or crawling up into lap on cue, providing a plausible excuse to leave.
- Dog may be trained to vocalize as if urgently needing to go outside, on cue.

Assist to Leave the Area by Finding Exit

Just as a guide dog can be taught to "Find the Exit" in a store or hotel lobby or a classroom, a number of persons with PTSD or panic disorder report it is helpful to have their service dogs schooled to lead them to the nearest Exit on command or cue, whenever they fear imminent loss of self control due to anger or experience symptoms that are precursors to a full blown panic attack or disassociative episode. The dog should learn ahead of time where a specific exit can be found, be encouraged to find it, rewarded for finding it with several practice sessions minimum in a new place before he can be expected to find it on command without a lot of help from the handler and/or a trainer. It can take months of schooling for this to become a reliable strategy for leaving an area when symptoms flare up, especially if the dog is expected to respond to symptoms as a cue rather than a verbal command. Input from trainers clarified the dog does not drag the person; the partner must be willing and able to immediately respond to the dog's effort to lead them away from a stressful situation as soon as the person feels a slight tug on the leash.

- Dog is schooled to find a specific exit to a classroom, an office, a store, a hotel lobby etc. on command or cue to assist someone to leave a high stress situation.

Provide Deep Pressure for Calming Effect

Those who suffer from panic attacks have reported that the pressure of the weight of a medium size dog or a large dog against their abdomen and chest has a significant calming effect. It can shorten the duration of the attack, often prevent the symptoms from escalating. This same task performed by service dogs for its calming benefit for children and adults who are autistic and prone to panic attacks has become known as "deep pressure therapy" in the assistance dog field. One way it is performed is to have a medium size dog lie atop someone who is lying on their back on a floor, bed or sofa, forepaws over the shoulders of the partner. A large dog could be too heavy in that position; also some dogs dislike it. A second way is have the partner sit up in a recliner chair, with the large dog approaching from the side so when he does a "Lap Up" on command, standing on his hind legs, he will be draping most of his body weight across the partner's abdomen, lying partly on his side, leaning his shoulder into the partner's torso, his forelegs on the other side of the partner's lap. Once trained to quietly hold that position for up to five minutes, this same task can be adapted to just about any chair, couch or bench seat his partner sits on. A dog should be given a rest break for at least a minute, back on all four paws, before repeating this task on his hind legs. Similarly, the weight and warmth of a medium to large size dog lying across the partner's lap, applying pressure to that person's stomach and chest, may be utilized in a vehicle's front seat, on the ground or in another location that supports the dog's entire body in the Down position, for as long as needed during a panic attack.

Dog is trained to provide deep pressure therapy during a panic attack. Precise behavior at such a time may be dictated by dog's size, preference and partner's location. Dog must be trained to promptly get Off the person on command.

Crowd Control, Panic Prevention In Public

A number of individuals disabled by PTSD and other psychiatric conditions report one of their difficulties in maintaining employment is the claustrophobic reaction they suffer when a colleague, boss, or customer comes too close to them.

The revulsion they experience is not limited to the workplace of course. Avoiding situations where closeness may take place will lead to someone becoming increasingly homebound. Through teamwork with a service dog, some of these individuals have regained the ability to do their own shopping and to ride on public transportation. Such teamwork may also enable them to cope better with the risk of close contact in the workplace or at a Little League game, the polls on election day and other places which may draw a crowd, helping the partner to lead a much more normal life.

Dog is first trained on how to brace himself on a Stand Stay so that he cannot be jostled out of position. Technique was developed by service dog trainers to protect patients with Reflex Sympathy Dystrophy from accidental bumps that can trigger an excruciatingly painful RSD flare-up. Same task can prevent or reduce panic by creating enough distance for a situation to become tolerable. A large sturdy dog is schooled to move into Position (front, behind, left or right side) and to brace for possible impact with an innocuous command, such as "Stay Close." Dog holds his ground, preventing people from making body contact with his partner while in line or on a bus, elevator or in the same room etc. Enhance the effectiveness of this strategy by asking a person to step back, using dog's alleged fear of having his paws stepped on as a plausible reason for making such a request.

- Dog is trained to repeatedly circle the partner to keep people at a comfortable distance. Short term strategy for backing people off.

- Dog of any size can be schooled to move fast into requested Position, usually in front of or behind the partner and perform a quick Down Stay. Must learn to drop with his back to the person approaching or persons in line. Should lie flat on his side or at least on one hip, to maximize the distance between the partner and nearest person. If worried a small dog might be stepped, have him do a Stand-Stay instead, with the tail end nearest to the person to be kept at bay so as to maximize the distance this achieves.

Arouse From Fear Paralysis or Disassociation Spell

In Parkinson's, where the person freezes and is unable move, the dog is schooled to assist the individual by making physical contact, such as lightly tapping the person's shoe with his paw. This apparently is sufficient to break the spell, allowing the individual to resume movement. Reportedly, similar behavior—physical stimulation through pawing or nose nudging—can rouse someone from a disassociation state, at least sufficiently to make the person aware of his/her plight, thus providing a chance to focus and fight the symptoms. This may also be effective in fear paralysis, another symptom of PTSD. Transforming it from an accidental spontaneous behavior into a reliable skill will require months of diligent schooling and practice. (Training Note: Simulate the trance state, then use click and treat or "Yes!" and treat to teach the dog the desired response, perhaps hiring a professional dog trainer to shape and reinforce the behavior. If there are frequent practice sessions in a variety of settings, this training may enable the dog to perform this valuable task whenever the freezing behavior, fear paralysis or disassociation occurs in real life. Alternatively, teach it as a hearing dog alert to a wristwatch alarm.) Those who lose awareness of the dog and their surroundings when disassociating should consider using a Waist Leash or type with a wrist band that can be velcroed to one's wrist so the dog won't wander off if you drop the leash when you disassociate outside your home.

- ~ Dog is trained to nudge handler during freezing behavior to rouse handler from a disassociative state or fear paralysis.
- ~ Dog is trained to respond with nudging and/or pawing whenever he hears the beeping from a wristwatch with an alarm clock function, which his partner can set to go off as frequently as desired, so the dog can arouse the seated or ambulating partner from a disassociative episode at home or in public. If fully alert, the partner can just reset the alarm before the alarm due to go off, unless he chooses to give the dog a practice session. Could be useful for someone with appointments or classes to get to or other responsibilities, if he or she is responsive to a service dog nudging or pawing when disassociating.

IV. Security Enhancement Tasks

Not every person who becomes the victim of assault develops a psychiatric disorder with symptoms severe enough to qualify them as disabled under the Americans With Disabilities Act. But those who do become disabled by Post Traumatic Stress Disorder (PTSD) experience the world as an extremely dangerous place. This psychological injury can be just as disabling as an injury which causes a loss of vision or hearing. It amputates the sense of safety or security that most people take for granted. The tasks in this section offer the human partner some innovative coping strategies. Teamwork with a service dog can empower the victim to win back a measure of independence and to resist incorrect and unrealistic responses. For the traumatized handler, a service dog who masters these tasks will be an invaluable ally.

Coping With Fear of Hidden Intruders in the Home

Assault victims who develop post traumatic stress disorder (PTSD) may find it extremely difficult to live alone or to spend time in the house when other household members are not at home for fear of being attacked again. Others are afraid to leave the house for fear of returning to discover there is a hidden intruder. A state of mind known as hyper vigilance, in which all senses are straining to detect where the next attack is coming from, is common to victims of assault who develop PTSD. It can impair the ability to function in a home or public setting. In addition, some of the tasks suggested here may help patients with sleep disturbances such as night terrors to cope better with the fear they experience.

Provide a Reality Check—Who's There?

PTSD hyper vigilance, hypnagogic hallucinations, flashbacks, nightmares, night terror or extreme sleep deprivation from Depression lead to distorted reality perceptions. One isn't always sure whether the voices in the other room or a certain noise is real or is part of the psychiatric disability. It can be tremendously reassuring if the service dog is trained to alert to anything unusual in the real environment. It is essential to hold practice sessions where by pre-arrangement, a friend approaches the house during the session or sneaks in quietly so he or she is standing in the next room when the dog is asked "Who's there?" Knowing how the dog behaves when there is a real cause for alarm can aid in interpreting his reaction at a later date, helping the partner decide whether to flee or relax.

Ask the service dog, "Who's There?" in excited tone of voice. The tone of voice and body language will encourage the dog to listen and to alert if need be. If nothing is there, the dog's initial interest will wane. He will relax and wander off to do something else.

To reduce fear an intruder may have entered the premises while the partner was out of the house, this "Who's There?" teamwork can also be utilized when returning home, upon entering the house. It can be immensely reassuring if the dog's body language indicates there are no unexpected visitors.

Strategies With a Portable Phone

The dog can be trained to bring a portable phone designated "for emergencies only" to any room in the house. While there are other reasons why this task could be a valuable one, in this particular case, the task could empower the handler to investigate a suspicious noise to hopefully lay her fears to rest, rather than flee the premises. The handler could keep a finger on the button pre programmed to dial 911 as a precaution. The handler also has the option of calling a friend and keeping the person on the line while checking out the premises. If returning home from an outing, the handler could have the dog enter the home and bring the portable phone to the front or back porch. It could even be delivered to the car if the dog utilizes a special doggy door with a lock keyed to an electronic key device on the dog's collar, if partner does not feel it would be safe to open the door for the dog or approach the porch or deck. This task could mitigate the handler's overpowering fear of going into the house after work or running errands and prevent the partner from becoming housebound.

- Dog trained to retrieve a portable phone and deliver it to any room in the house so partner can investigate a suspicious noise, with friend on the line or 911 available.
- Dog can be trained to enter the home through a doggy door or another entrance, to fetch the phone and deliver it to the partner who is waiting outside or in car to use it.

Call for Help in Advance

Having a friend listen via speaker phone to everything that goes on in the house from the moment the handler enters the premises gives extra insurance that police will soon be on their way if it turns out the handler's fear of a hidden intruder was justified. The dog can be sent to depress the three inch wide white button that dials a pre programmed number on the K-9 Rescue Phone before the handler steps foot in the house. Also a service dog could be sent in the middle of the night to operate the device before the handler leaves the bedroom. If a sympathetic support system is available, this option can help the handler resist calling the police every time he or she hears a strange noise or experiences a feeling of dread upon returning home. The K-9 Rescue phone remains functional in a power failure as it is equipped with a 21 day battery.

Dog trained to go to the location of the K-9 Rescue phone and push the large button to dial 911 or another pre-set number

BEFORE partner enters the home. If anything dreadful occurs when the partner goes inside, it will be heard by the 911 operator or a friend over the speaker-phone, so help can be sent fast.

Same task, but performed from a different location, requiring the dog to be trained to habitually follow a specific route from the bedroom or other designated rooms to the place where the K-9 Rescue Phone is waiting for the dog to operate it.

Lighting Up Dark Rooms

A service dog can be trained to precede the handler into rooms, hallways or the basement, turning on lamps or overhead lights to reduce the partner's fear of a lurking intruder, when a strange noise or some other stimulus necessitates inspection of the home before the partner can resume daily life activities or go back to sleep. A floor pedal device, a touch lamp device for lamps with a metal base or inexpensive wireless lights to illuminate dark areas if a dog nudges them are some of the clever options available if worried about wall scratches from the dog pawing conventional light switches. A touch pad made for the severely disabled could control up to six lights at once throughout the house and be operated by a service dog.

When the team arrives home after dark, the service dog's ability to operate a touch lamp or other devices can be put to good use to mitigate the partner's fear of returning home to a hidden intruder. The dog can be trained to enter a dark residence by himself to switch on one or more lamps. Not only is the light itself beneficial, the dog's behavior during the performance of the task will provide reality based feedback to aid the handler in the decision of whether or not to risk entering the house. If somebody did happen to be inside, chances are very high the dog will skip the task or rush off to investigate the new scent as soon as he performs the task. This teamwork approach is an option for a victim of assault that is arguably superior to relying on a timer to turn on the lights when the sun goes down.

- Dog must learn to operate light switches and/or other devices like a floor pedal device or touch lamps. Then the dog is schooled to precede handler into each room turning on lights one by one to reduce partner's fear of a lurking intruder.

- Dog is trained to enter a dark home or apartment by himself to switch on lamp(s) to reduce the partner's fear of entering the premises.

Assist with Escape Strategies: Open Front Door

One option to increase safety before responding to suspicious sounds is to routinely send the dog to open the front door on command, if there is a storm door to prevent him from running off. The dog's behavior during this task will serve as "a reality check," helping the partner to discern if anyone is waiting down the hall or in another room. The partner can then escape using another route if there is a real reason to do so. (Training Note: start at front door, move back to room(s) only 5 ft. per week to build up confidence before adding more distance, to ingrain a route from the door to each room. This is how to achieve reliability on any "place command.") If fear drove partner to exit without sending the dog to front door, the dog can be trained to assist the partner to get back inside.

The dog is trained to open the front door by tugging on a strap attached to a lever handle installed on the interior side of the Front Door. Secondly, the dog must learn to go from the bedroom and /or other rooms all the way to the front door to perform the task on command, at any time of day or night.

The dog could be trained to open a locked door from the inside on command by tugging on a strap attached to a lever handle. This could enable his partner who exited by a window or another route, to get back inside without needing to wake up a sleeping family member or call a locksmith.

Fear Management In Public

These tasks for working with a service dog in public settings gives a victim of assault new coping strategies that could go a long way to mitigating the disabling fear experienced as a consequence of the trauma. At the same time, if utilized correctly, none of these tasks will spoil a service dog's gentle trusting nature.

Reducing Hyper-Vigilance Through Teamwork

Victims of assault who develop disabling PTSD report success in coping with their highly fearful state of mind, called hyper vigilance, through teamwork with a service dog. The dog selected should have a laid back, amiable, very confident temperament. The dog must be well socialized so he can handle the challenges of public access work in a calm manner. He must be trained to remain obedient and unobtrusive even if the handler reacts with extreme terror to various stimuli, seeing potential threats where none exist. By remaining calm in such situations, the service dog's relaxed confident demeanor serves as a reality check for one whose perception of danger can no longer be trusted. This enables hyper vigilant individuals to more accurately assess the situation and to make reality informed decisions about what to do. Like guide dog and hearing dog handlers who rely on their dogs' body language to enhance their ability to safely navigate their environment, individuals with PTSD report impressive gains in their ability to function outside the home, relying on their dog's training and body language to compensate for the mental impairment they must contend with. Dog may also be taught to do a "Who's There?" reality check on command before entering a parking lot or other feared locations. (NOTE: When the approach of a jogger or some other innocent bystander triggers the handler's hyper vigilant fear she is in mortal danger, the last thing in the world that is needed is a fiercely protective guard dog who due to instinct or training leaps to the handler's defense with a frightening display of aggressive behavior. Such a reaction won't mitigate the disability by decreasing the victim's hyper vigilant state of mind. Rather it forces the handler to become much more vigilant, knowing this dog is capable of hurting any human whom he perceives to be a threat to the team. Trying to deal with the dog's hyper vigilance as well as your own will be counter productive and exhausting. Furthermore, aggressive acting dogs do not qualify for access as legitimate service animals. Much more could be said on the subject, but suffice it to say, this would be a misguided and dangerous approach to helping assault victims cope with psychiatric disorders like PTSD.)

Keep Suspicious Strangers Away

A dog is a much better crime deterrent than burglar alarms, extra locks and security lighting according to police statistics. Those who wish to enhance the psychological deterrent effect should consider the dog's size, color and breed appearance in making a selection. Studies have revealed people are much more afraid of black dogs than light colored ones. By way of example, a large black Labrador Retriever will have the same gentle temperament but look twice as formidable as a yellow Labrador Retriever. A Great Dane is going to be more of a deterrent than a toy poodle.

This segment describes four tasks which could assist a handler to keep suspicious strangers at bay. However, the tasks are only meant to create an illusion. The dog must be rigorously schooled NOT to be protective in these situations even if partner acts fearful. A service dog should only perform these tasks to please his handler and/or earn a treat.

Actual protection training /attack training is ethically prohibited for legitimate service dogs. A service dog should never be allowed to bark AT strangers in public. The following tasks will provide much safer and much more useful kinds of behavior in the long run than having an over protective dog. These tasks offer a non-violent alternative to carrying a weapon for someone coping with the fear of another assault. Useful as a bluff strategy for other kinds of assistance dogs too. Won't ruin the underlying good natured tolerance for strangers that is the appropriate temperament every assistance dog should exhibit and be tested for prior to any training. (Note: Please do not publicize the fact that some assistance dog handlers may teach their dogs bluff tasks for this could have a detrimental impact on the safety of a team. However, it would be honest and acceptable to say to a reporter or write: "Service dogs can be schooled to perform tasks that enhance the safety of their disabled owners." Realize that it is never acceptable to alarm the public, arousing fear of assistance dogs when addressing this topic in a public forum. This is a very thin line that must be walked with great sensitivity.)

The dog is trained to obey the bluff command "Cover Me." Dog learns to jump up and turn around, standing next to his partner, facing backwards. (It is a Stand-stay obedience exercise with a dog facing in a different direction than usual. A mugger may receive the impression the dog is watching for trouble.)

May also train a dog to turn his head from side to side, while facing people behind you. Taught by using click and treat or verbal "Yes" and treat, rewarding him whenever he turns head to the left. Use the bluff command: "Watch My Back." Psychologically, with a large dog, it's a crime deterrent, while partner operates an ATM machine or while quickly unlocking a car or an office door. Dog does not actually do anything more than hold a Stand-stay position, while giving the impression that he is visually scanning the area for possible trouble. After the dog turns his head from side to side, four to six times in a row, reward him, then ask him to repeat it.

Dog rises from a Down-stay position to assume a Stand-stay position next to or in front of his disabled partner. What changes this from a routine obedience exercise to an effective illusion is teaching the dog to spring up quickly when the handler uses a bluff command such as, "On Guard!" To heighten the illusion, the handler should grip the dog's collar as if the dog needs to be restrained from charging forward.

Dog is taught to "Bark for Help," on command, or when you snap your fingers, to earn a treat. This vocalizing attracts attention to the team, scaring off a mugger or some other predator, for the last thing a criminal wants is the public's attention focused on his activities. Teaching the dog to bark enthusiastically, instead of falling silent in eager anticipation of his treat after only two or three barks requires several months of schooling in the home, vehicle and a variety of other locations, before it will be a dependable task.

Increase Safety in Public, at ATM With Equipment, and Teamwork

Criminals are not certain how a service dog might react if a stranger tries to steal something out of his backpacks, something that can work to the team's advantage. Many mobility impaired handlers put their wallet, other valuables and ID in a service dog's backpacks for safe keeping, as there has not been a case of a service dog being mugged since their inception over a quarter century ago. While having the dog wear backpacks is not considered a task, per se, it could allow victims of assault and others with a psychiatric disability to substantially reduce their vulnerability as a potential target for purse snatchers, pickpockets and muggers. If the individual has flashbacks, disassociative episodes or becomes disorientated, the backpacks may prevent others from taking advantage of the individual at such times. Ethical guidelines puts the amount of weight a dog can carry at 15% of the dog's total body weight. The 15% includes the weight of the harness with empty backpacks, about 2 to 4 pounds, depending on its design. By working together at an ATM and check out stands, a handler with a large service dog can minimize any appearance of vulnerability and conceal the amount of cash he or she is carrying, reducing the stress associated with performing this high anxiety chore for a victim of assault.

Dog trained to work cooperatively with the handler at an ATM machine, by obediently doing a "Paws up" and "Stay," to allow the card and checks to be removed from backpack or to permit the cash dispensed by an ATM to be discretely returned to the backpack. It enables a handler to remain in an upright position, blocking ATM's screen from view, rather than making self much more vulnerable to a mugging by bending down to fumble with the backpack zipper or velcro tabs. DISCLAIMER: Please understand this is NOT a task that will legally "count" as a trained task acceptable in a court of law as proof the dog meets the legal definition of a service animal. It is simply an optional extra, a "bonus aid," which any dog lover, disabled or non disabled, may enjoy. Such items could be carried in a purse or fanny pack, so it is a matter of personal choice.

Author: Joan Froling; Copyright on original Task List February 1, 1998. Copyrighted this updated version on July 30, 2009. Contact author for reprint permission: *www.sterlingservicedogs.org* May not be published or reproduced in part or in its entirety without reprint permission.

Permission to reprint granted by Joan Froling, September 3, 2009.

Appendix 7

On October 5, 2005, *The Chronicle-Telegram*, Wellington and Oberlin, Ohio, newspaper published "Paws and Take a Deep Breath" by Stephen Szucs, focusing on Jane Miller's work with Psychiatric Service Dogs. See page 226 to read the article. Permission to reprint the article granted August 13, 2009.

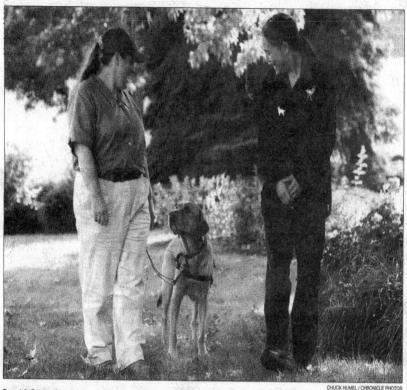

CHUCK HUMEL / CHRONICLE PHOTOS

Tracy, left, Baron, a therapy dog, and clinical social worker Jane Miller. Tracy half-joked, "Baron gave me a new leash on life. He makes it possible for me to get up and face each day." Tracy has been diagnosed with post-traumatic stress disorder.

Paws and take a deep breath

Social worker says dogs are therapeutic

Stephen Szucs
The Chronicle-Telegram

When clinical social worker Jane Miller works with those dealing with mental health issues, she tries to give them a new leash on life.

Miller, a 25-year resident of Oberlin, coincidentally learned the importance of a psychiatric service dog, after watching her own dog, Umaya, interact with clients in her office waiting room.

Miller, whose previous office used to be in Cleveland Heights, brought cancer stricken Umaya into the office after the dog had received radiation treatments.

"I didn't have time to drive her home after treatment and before I had to go to work, so I brought her to the office," Miller said. "Umaya didn't look well, but she glowed with energy and walked around visiting with everyone."

When Umaya accompanied Miller in therapy sessions, Miller noticed the added comfort the dog brought to her clients.

She said the dog often allowed them to relax and talk about what they had a hard time discussing.

"Umaya really transformed the therapeutic process for me," Miller said. "If a client began to cry, Umaya would be there by them, and they would pet her and continue to talk. Over time, clients would be saying to me, 'I need an Umaya.'"

Miller would eventually meet Tracy, a client who had been diagnosed with post-traumatic stress disorder, and was suffering through depression and anxiety.

"When I first met Jane, I couldn't even function as a human being," Tracy said. "I had trouble putting words together into a sentence, and difficulty talking with anyone. I couldn't even leave my house."

Miller worked with Tracy, while Umaya comforted her through her sessions. After a careful assessment, Miller thought a psychiatric service dog would make a nice fit for Tracy.

"You have to make sure the client is able to take care of the dog while taking care of themselves," Miller said. "It's really an added responsibility, but sometimes that's what the person needs."

Tracy had already owned three dogs, but none of which could be trained for her disorder.

She was paired with a golden Labrador retriever named, Baron, who would be trained to react to Tracy and certain situations. Whether she's crying or spending too much time in bed, Baron's been trained to gently paw at her.

"I never could eat in a restaurant before Baron," Tracy said. "Baron will lie across my feet, and sort of anchors me there. He helps to keep me calm and centered."

Baron also helps to keep Tracy composed in countertop transactions at a bank or store, where he's been trained to press up against her.

Miller has worked with a number of clients like Tracy, assessing them for psychiatric service dogs and guiding them through the process.

Miller said it makes a lot of sense that dogs can be trained to change our lives.

"For many who don't have anyone to rely on, a dog helps to teach them unconditional love," Miller said.

Abbreviations

AAA = Animal Assisted Activities

AAT = Animal Assisted Therapy

AD = Assistance Dog

ADA = Americans With Disabilities Act

ADI = Assistance Dog International

AKC = American Kennel Club

APDT = Association of Pet Dog Trainers

CADO = Coalition of Assistance Dog Organizations

CCI = Canine Companions for Independence

CDBC = Certified Dog Behavioral Consultant

CGC = AKC sponsored Canine Good Citizen Test

C&T= Click and Treat

CPDT = Certified Pet Dog Trainer

DBSA = Depression and Bipolar Support Alliance

DOJ = Department of Justice

ESA = Emotional Support Animal

IAABC = International Association of Animal Behavioral Consultants

IAADP = International Association of Assistance Dog Partners

LISW = Licensed Independent Social Worker

NAMI = National Alliance of Mental Illness

NEADS = National Education of Assistance Dog Services

OT = Owner Trained

PAT = Public Access Test through the Assistance Dog International

PBB = Puppies Behind Bars

PSD = Psychiatric Service Dog

PSDIT = Psychiatric Service Dog in Training

PTSD = Posttraumatic Stress Disorder

PWD = Person with Disability

SD = Service Dog

SDIT = Service Dog in Training

TADI = The Assistance Dog Institute

TDI = Therapy Dog International

TDInc. = Therapy Dog Incorporated

UKC = United Kennel Club

Glossary

Assistance Dog: A generic term for guide, hearing, or service dog specifically trained to do more than one task to mitigate the effects of an individual's disability. The presence of a dog for protection, personal defense, or comfort does not qualify that dog as an assistance dog.

Assistance Dog Instructor: A person affiliated with a program who is recognized by that program as being directly responsible for educating an assistance dog team and/or meeting other educational requirements of the program.

Assistance Dog Trainer: A person affiliated with a program as being directly responsible for the training and conduct of an assistance dog in training.

Client: Any individual who is an applicant, student, or graduate of an assistance dog program.

Facility Dog: A specially trained dog that is working with a volunteer or professional who is trained by a program. The work of a facility dog can include visitations or professional therapy in one or more locations. Public access is permitted only when the dog and handler, who is a trained volunteer or professional, is directly working with a client with a disability.

Hearing Dog: A dog that alerts individuals who are deaf or hard of hearing to specific sounds.

Privately Trained Assistance Dog: An assistance dog trained by an individual who is not affiliated with an assistance dog training program.

Program: An organization involved in the training of assistance dogs.

Public Access: The right of a person with a disability to be accompanied by his/her assistance dog in all public accommodations. Public access is granted to the person with the disability, not to the assistance dog.

Public Access for Assistance Dog Instructors and Assistance Dog Trainers: The ability of an assistance dog trainer to work with a dog in public places in order to replicate rather than simulate real life situations.

Puppy raiser: A person or family appointed by a program to socialize and prepare a young dog to enter formal training.

Service Dog: A dog that works for individuals with disabilities other than blindness or deafness. They are trained to perform a wide variety of tasks including but not limited to; pulling a wheelchair, bracing, retrieving, alerting to a medical crisis, and providing assistance in a medical crisis.

Permission granted by the Assistance Dog International, Inc. to reprint the ADI Glossary of Terms from Website: *www.assistancedogsinternational.org.*

Level Double-A Conformance to Web Content Accessibility Guidelines 1.0

Section 508 Compliant

Additional terms referred to in this book*

Psychiatric Service Dogs: A service dog trained individually to mitigate the effects of their disabled partner's psychiatric disabilities by performing specific tasks.

Psychiatric Service Dogs in Training: A service dog trained individually to mitigate the effects of their disabled partner's psychiatric disabilities that is not completely trained in public access and task trained.

Handler or Partner: In this book refers to the disabled individual that cares for his/her PSD.

Therapy Dog: An individual's pet which has been trained, tested, certified and insured to work in hospitals, libraries, schools, and other institutional settings. (See Appendix for Delta Society, TD Inc., and TDI for certification programs.) The therapy dog and partner visit facilities to provide comfort, stress reduction, emotional support, and companionship. Therapy dogs are not service dogs. Service dogs work for their disabled handler whereas therapy dogs are trained to help groups of people in various settings.

An example of a therapy dog was Umaya who was Jane's co-therapist and went to work with her every day. Simcha and Ahava, Jane's two Golden Retrievers have followed Umaya's lead and are now Jane's therapy dogs that go to work with her every day as her co-therapists.

*Additional terms written by: Jane Miller and not part of the ADI glossary.

Resources

Introduction
General Information About Working Dogs:

Becker, Marty. *The Healing Power of Pets: Harnessing the Ability of Pets to Make and Keep People Happy and Healthy*. New York: Hyperion, 2002.

Bondarenko, Nina. *Hearts, Minds and Paws: A Book on Dogs and Working Dogs*. UK: Aeneas, 2007.

Davis, Marcie, and Melissa Bunnell. *Working Like Dogs: The Service Dog Guidebook*. Minneapolis: Alpine Publications, 2007.

Mehus-Roe, Kristin. *Working Dogs: True Stories of Dogs and Their Handlers*. New York: BowTie, 2003.

Nye, Julie. *Practical Partners: A Service Dog Research Guide*. New York: Fieldstone-Hill, 2005.

Sakson, Sharon. *Paws & Effect: The Healing Power of Dogs*. New York: Alyson Books, 2007.

Warshauer, Sherry Bennett. *Everyday Heroes: Extraordinary Dogs Among Us*. New York: Howell Book House, 1998.

General Websites About Working Dogs:

www.associationofanimalbehaviorprofessionals.com (see glossary and Abbreviations)

www.assistancedogsinternational.org/

www.deltasociety.org

http://healing-companions.com (the author, Jane Miller's Website)

Helper dogs—Education and Support for People and Service Dogs see:

http://herizenfyre-ivil.tripod.com:80

International Association of Assistance Dog Partners see:

www.iaadp.org

www.k9events.com/EtiquetteforSDHandlers.pdf

landofpuregold.com/service.htm

www.petsandpeople.org

http://servicedogcentral.org/

www.shoreservicedogs.com (see history of service dogs)

www.supportpartnersprogram.com

www.tamaractollers.com (Nancy Tucker, contributor to the book)

General Assistance Dog Yahoo Groups:

Search Yahoo! Groups for Assistance Dogs; see "Operant Conditioning Assistance Dogs," "Owner Trained Assistance Dogs," and "Assistance Dogs," as helpful groups to join. See:

assistance-dogs@yahoogroups.com

OC-Assist-Dogs@yahoogroups.com

OT-ServiceDogs@yahoogroups.com

Personal Stories About Working Dogs:

Goldstein, Bruce. *Puppy Chow Is Better than Prozac: The True Story of a Man and the Dog Who Saved His Life.* New York: Da Capo, 2008.

Lingenfelter, Mike, and David Frei. *The Angel by My Side: The True Story of a Dog Who Saved a Man...and a Man Who Saved a Dog.* New York: Hay House, 2002.

Ogden, Paul. *Chelsea: The Story of a Signal Dog.* New York: Fawcett, 1993.

Therapy Dog Resources:

Butler, Kris. *Therapy Dogs Today: Their Gifts, Our Obligation.* Grand Rapids: Funpuddle Associates, 2004.

Davis, Kathy Diamond. *Therapy Dogs: Training Your Dog to Reach Others.* Grand Rapids: Dogwise, 2002.

Kruger, Katherine A., Symme W. Trachtenberg, and James A. Serpell. *Can Animals Help Humans Heal? Animal-Assisted Interventions in Adolescent Mental Health.* Center for the Interaction of Animals and Society, University of Pennsylvania School of Veterinary Medicine, July 2004.

Therapy Dog Websites: *www.deltasociety.org*
Therapy Dogs International see: *www.tdi-dog.org*
Therapy Dogs Incorporated see: *www.therapydogs.com*

Chapter 2: Canine Rx: Finding the Right Companion
Americans with Disabilities Act Resources:

Stefan, Susan. *Unequal Rights: Discrimination Against People With Mental Disabilities and the Americans With Disabilities Act*. Washington, DC: American Psychological Association, 2001.

Americans with Disabilities Act Websites:
www.ada.gov
ADA Business BRIEF: Service Animals
www.ada.gov/svcanimb.htm
www.ada-audio.org/Archives/
www.adawatch.org
www.bazelon.org (see disability rights resources)
www.disabilityadvocates.us (see ADA amendment act of 2008)

Equal Employment Opportunity Commission see:
www.eeoc.gov (see ADA law and government policy)

Job Accommodation Network see: *http://janweb.icdi.wvu.edu/*

National Empowerment Center see:
www.power2u.org/
www.thomas.gov (for federal legislative information)

United States Department of Justice see: *www.usdoj.go*

Breed Resources:
Hoffman, Martha. *Lend Me an Ear: The Temperament, Selection and Training of the Hearing Ear Dog*. Grand Rapids: Doral, 1999.

Tortora, Daniel F. *Right Dog For You. New York: Fireside*, 1983.
"Breed Types: What's In a Name" by Micky Niego (see appendix)
Selecting Canine Candidates for Working Careers DVD/CD Set
by Dee Ganley and Barbara Handelman (2006).

Breed Websites:
Animal Kennel Club see: *www.akc.org (see breed information)*
www.darnfar.com
www.dogbreedinginfo.com
www.iaadp.org (see breed information, article on the "Quest for the Suitable Adult Candidate" and article about health screening)

United Kennel Club see:
www.ukcdogs.com (see breed information)
www.yourpurebredpuppy.com/

Temperament Testing Websites:
Assistance Dogs International, Inc. see:
www.adionline.org (see public access test)
American Temperament Test Society, Inc. see:
www.atts.org (see sample temperament test)
International Association of Assistance Dog Partners see:
www.iaadp.org (see sample temperament test)
www.k9events.com (see socialization checklist)
American Veterinary Society of Animal Behavior see:
www.avsabonline.org (see puppy socialization)
www.diamondsintheruff.com (see puppy socialization)
www.paw-rescue.org (dog tips- temperament)
www.puppyprodigies.org

Volhard Puppy Aptitude Test see:
www.volhard.com/pages/pat.php

Articles About Contributors to the Book:
www.cbsnews.com/stories/2000/02/23/48hours/main164225.shtml?source=search_story
www.villagevoice.com/1999-12-28/news/scout-s-honor/

Chapter 3: Prison Puppies Free Veterans from Combat Veterans' Stories:

Kopelman, Jay. *From Baghdad to America: Life Lessons from a Dog Named Lava.* Skyhorse, 2003.

Kopelman, Jay. *From Baghdad, With Love: A Marine, the War, and a Dog Named Lava.* Lyons, 2008.

Assistance Dog Organizations:
Bergin University of Canine Studies—Paws For Purple Hearts: *www.berginu.org/academics/PPH.html*
Canine Companions For Independence see: *www.cci.org*
www.freedomdogs.org
National Education for Assistance Dog Services see: *www.neads.org*
Puppies Behind Bars see: *www.puppiesbehindbars.com*

Veteran's Websites:
www.cominghomeproject.net
Iraq and Afghanistan Veterans of America see: *www.iava.org*
Charity for Military Sexual Trauma see: *www.packparachute.org/*
Program for Anxiety & Traumatic Stress Studies see: *www.patss.com*

The PTSD Help Network see: *www.ptsdhelp.net*
National Center for PTSD Home see: *www.ptsd.va.gov*
www.thetowerofhope.org/
Veterans and Families see: *www.veteransandfamilies.org*
www.vetwow.com
Welcome To Vietnam Veterans of America see: *www.vva.org*

Articles About Veterans:
www.abcnews.go.com (see Iraq Vet Gets Dog, New Chance at Life)
www.azcentral.com (see Program Pairs War Vets, Dogs)
www.cnn.com (see Dogs Chase Nightmares of War Away)
www.fetchdog.com (see Q & A with Bill Campbell)
www.magnumphotos.com (see Wounded Veteran Raymond Hubbard)
www.nytimes.com/ (see "After Combat, Victims of an Inner War," "Prison Puppies," "Veterans Helped by Healing Paws," and "Veterans Affairs Faces Surge of Disability Claims")
www.projo.com (see 2 Puppies Report for Duty at R.I. Veterans Home to be Trained to Assist Disabled Vets)
http://online.wsj.com (see Sit! Stay! Snuggle!: An Iraq Vet Finds His Dog Tuesday)
http://video.on.nytimes.com:80/?fr_story=1c19a2e38f08b1b 1bbb7e54c837485938cbc401c&excamp=NYT-E-I-NYT-E-AT-0604-L7&WT.mc_ev=click&WT.mc_id=

PTSD Resource:
Naparstek, Belleruth. *Invisible Heroes: Survivors of Trauma and How They Heal.* New York: Bantam, 2004.

PTSD and Mental Health Websites:
American Psychiatric Association: *www.psych.org/*
www.bipolar.about.com

Depression and Bipolar support Alliance see:
www.dbsalliance.org
www.everydayhealth.com (see health benefits of dogs)
Guided Imagery and Meditation Resources by Belleruth Naparstek see: *www.healthjourneys.com*
International Association of Assistance Dog Partners see: *www.iaadp.org* (see PSD tasks)
National Alliance of Mental Illness see: *www.nami.org*
National Mental Health Association: *www.nmha.org/*
Department of Health & Human Services see:
www.ncbi.nlm.nih.gov/ (look up any research for articles and information)

Psych Central: *www.psychcentral.com/*
Mental Health Article: *www.mentalhelp.net/poc/view_doc php?type=doc&id=14844&cn=109*

PTSD Research:
For those interested in the science behind what may be occurring, Dr. Porge's, polyvagal theory may provide a neurophysiological explanation of how PSDs frequently inhibit feelings of anxiety and panic. (see: Porges SW. 1995. Orienting in a defensive world: Mammalian modifications of our evolutionary heritage. A Polyvagal Theory. <u>Psychophysiology</u> 32:301-318. or *www.nexuspub.com/articles/2006/interview_ma.htm* for more details.)

In conclusion, those with psychiatric disabilities benefit considerably by having a service dog. Natalie Sachs-Erickson et al. noted in their study (see: Sachs-Ericsson, N. J., Hansen, N., Fitzgerald, S. (2002). Benefits of Assistance Dogs: A review. Rehabilitation Psychology, 47(3), 251–277.) that, " through clinical observation, anecdotal reports, and retrospective and cross-sectional studies, preliminary support was found for the conclusion that ADs (assistance dogs) have a positive impact on individuals' health, psychological well-being, social interactions, performance of activities, and participation in various life roles at home and in the community" (2002). For anyone interested in reading some of these studies they can find the abstracts and articles on the Delta Societies website (see: *www.deltasociety.org*, see healthy reasons to have a pet) and the brochure "The Health Benefits of Companion Animals" provides citations and a brief summary of the research at *www.pawssf.org/*) also see safe pet guide.

Chapter 4: Sit, Stay Soothe: Training Your New Companion Training Resources:

Aloff, Brenda. *Get Connected With Your Dog. Emphasizing the Relationship While Training Your Dog.* Dogwise, 2008.

Clothier, Suzanne. *Bones Would Rain From the Sky: Deepening Our Relationships with Dogs.* Grand Rapids: Grand Central, 2002.

Dunbar, Ian. *Dog Behavior: An Owner's Guide to a Happy Healthy Pet.* New York: Howell Book House, 1999.

Fogle, Bruce. *The Dog's Mind: Understanding Your Dog's Behavior (Howell Reference Books).* New York: Howell Book House, 1992.

Ganley, Dee. *Changing People Changing Dogs: Positive Solutions for Difficult Dogs.* Dees Dogs, 2008.

McConnell, Patricia B., and Aimee M. Moore. *Family Friendly Dog Training: A Six Week Program for You and Your Dog.* McConnell, 2007.

Miller, Pat. *The Power of Positive Dog Training.* New York: Wiley, 2001.

Owens, Paul and Norma Eckrote. *The Dog Whisperer: A Compassionate, Nonviolent Approach to Dog Training*. New York: Adams Media Corporation, 1999.

Rugaas, Turid. *My Dog Pulls. What Do I Do?* Grand Rapids: Dogwise, 2005.

Ryan, Terry. *Coaching People to Train Their Dogs*. Chicago: Legacy Canine Behavior and Training, 2005.

Stilwell, Victoria. *It's Me or the Dog: How to Have the Perfect Pet It's Me or the Dog: How to Have the Perfect Pet*. New York: Hyperion, 2007.

UltimatePuppy. *The Ultimate Puppy Toolkit: A Complete, Fun, Step-By-Step Guide to Raising a Happy, Well-Adjusted Dog*. Premier Pet Products, 2005.

Weinberg, Dani. *Teaching People Teaching Dogs*. New York: Howln Moon, 2006.

Yin, Sophia A. *How to Behave So Your Dog Behaves*. Minneapolis: TFH Publications, 2004.

Training Websites and Videos:

Advanced Canine Behavior Seminar. By Patricia McConnell. Tawzer Dog Videos, 2001. DVD.

A Dog Training Video: Teamwork for People with Disabilities I & II. By Lydia Kelley and Stewart Nordensson. Top Dog Productions, 2003. DVD.

Teamwork & Teamwork II:

Service Dog training books, tapes, and videos *www.topdogusa.org/*

Sue Ailsby's training levels see:

www.dragonflyllama.com:80/%20DOGS/%20Dog1/levels.html

www.clickersolutions.com:80/

Vancouver Island Assistance Dogs see:

www.viassistancedogs.blogspot.com/

Schools for Training Trainers:

www.assistancedog.org/ (Bonnie Bergin's University)

Clicker Training:

Alexander, Melissa C. Click for Joy! Questions and Answers from Clicker Trainers and Their Dogs. Waltham: Sunshine Books, 2003.

Parsons, Emma. Click to Calm: Healing the Aggressive Dog. New York: Sunshine Books, 2004.

Pryor, Karen. Clicker Training For Dogs. Waltham: Sunshine Books, 2002.

Spector, Morgan. Clicker Training for Obedience: Shaping Top Performance-Positively. Waltham: Sunshine Books, 1999.

Clicker Train Your Own Assistance Dog. Prod. Barbara Handelman. Dog Training at Home, 2004. DVD.

Websites to Find a Trainer:

www.animalbehaviorcollege.com

www.animalbehaviorcounselors.org

Association of Pet Dog Trainers see: *www.apdt.com*

Certification Council For Professional Dog Trainers see: *www.ccpdt.org, www.dogpro.org*

The International Association of Animal Behavior Consultants see: *www.iaabc.org*

National K-9 Dog Trainers Association see: *www.nk9dta.com*

The National Association of Dog Obedience Instructors see: *www.nadoi.org*

www.trulydogfriendly.com

Chapter 6: Dogs Have Issues Too: Helping Your Dog Cope With Stress:

Ethics Resources:

Fine, Aubrey H. *Handbook on Animal-Assisted Therapy: Theoretical Foundations and Guidelines for Practice.* 1st ed. San Diego: Academic, 2000. quoted chapter 2

Iannuzzi, Dorothea and Rowan, Andrew. *Ethical Issues in Animal-Assisted Therpay Programs.* Anthrozoos. 4(30:154-163. 1991.

Ethics Websites:

www.assistancedogsinternational.org
Delta Society with their Minimum Standards for Service Dogs see: *www.DeltaSociety.org*
www.greenacreskennel.com (See Brambell's Five Freedoms)
www.vetpurdue.edu (see Alan Beck)

Stress and Canine Body Language Resources:

Aloff, Brenda. *Canine Body Language: A Photographic Guide—Interpreting the Native Language of the Domestic Dog.* Grand Rapids: Dogwise, 2005.

Arthur, Nan Kene. *Chill Out Fido!: How to Calm Your Dog.* Dogwise, 2008

Hallgren, Anders. *The ABC's of Dog Language. Dog House*, 1997.

Handelman, Barbara. *Canine Behavior: A Photo Illustrated Handbook.* Woof and Word, 2008.

Rugaas, Turid. *Barking: The Sound of a Language.* Dogwise, 2008.

Rugaas, Turid. *On Talking Terms With Dogs Calming Signals*. Lincolnwood: Legacy By Mail, 1997.

Sapolsky, Robert M. *Why Zebras Don't Get Ulcers, Third Edition*. New York: Holt Paperbacks, 2004.

Scholz, Martina, and Clarissa Von Reinhardt. *Stress in Dogs*. Grand Rapids: Dogwise, 2006.

Williams, Marta. *Learning Their Language: Intuitive Communication with Animals and Nature*. Chicago: New World Library, 2003.

Stress and Canine Body Language Websites & DVDs:

www.canineevents.com

www.diamondsintherough.com

Calming Signals: *What Your Dog Tells You*. By Turid Rugaas. Dogwise DVD, 2000. DVD.

Dog Talk: Understanding Canine Body Language and Communication. By Donna Duford. Tawzer Online Videos, 2006. DVD.

The Human-Animal Bond and Science Resources:

Beck, Alan M. *Between Pets and People: The Importance of Animal Companionship*. West Lafayette: Purdue UP, 1996.

Bekoff, Marc. *The Emotional Lives of Animals: A Leading Scientist Explores Animal Joy, Sorrow, and Empathy and Why They Matter*. Novato: New World Library, 2007.

Coren, Stanley. *How to Speak Dog: Mastering the Art of Dog-Human Communication*. New York: Free, 2000.

Goodall, Jane, and Marc Bekoff. *The Ten Trusts: What We Must Do to Care for The Animals We Love*. San Francisco: HarperSanFrancisco, 2002.

Grandin, Temple. *Animals in Translation: Using the Mysteries of Autism to Decode Animal Behavior.* New York: Scribner, 2005.

Hediger, Heini. *Psychology and Behaviour of Animals in Zoos and Circuses.* New York: Dover Publications, 1968.

Knapp, Caroline. *Pack of Two: The Intricate Bond Between People and Dogs.* Delta, 1999.

McConnell, Patricia B. *For the Love of a Dog: Understanding Emotion in You and Your Best Friend.* New York: Ballantine Books, 2006.

McElroy, Susan Chernak. *Animals as Guides for the Soul: Stories of Life-Changing Encounters.* New York: Wellspring/Ballantine, 1999.

Proctor, Pam, and Allen M. Schoen. *Love, Miracles, and Animal Healing: A Heartwarming Look at the Spiritual Bond Between Animals and Humans.* New York: Fireside, 1996.

Schoen, Allen M. *Kindred Spirits: How the Remarkable Bond Between Humans and Animals Can Change the Way we Live.* New York: Broadway, 2002.

Shanley, Karen. *Dogs of Dreamtime: A Story About Second Chances and the Power of Love.* Guilford, Conn: Lyons, 2005.

Smith, Cheryl. *The Rosetta Bone: The Key to Communication Between Humans and Canines.* New York: Howell Book House, 2004.

Williams, Marta. *Learning Their Language: Intuitive Communication with Animals and Nature.* Chicago: New World Library, 2003.

The Human-Animal Bond and Science Website and DVD:
www.drschoen.com (Allen Schoen's Website)
For the Love of a Dog: The Biology of Emotion in Two
     Species. Prod. Patricia McConnell. Tawzer Dog
     Videos, 2006. DVD.

Resources for Canine Health:
American National Red Cross. Dog First Aid. Yardley: Stay
     Well, 2007. Print.
Kay, Nancy. *Speaking for Spot: Be the Advocate Your Dog Needs
     to Live a Happy, Healthy, Longer Life.* Trafalgar Square
     Books, 2008.
Messonnier, Shawn. *Natural Health Bible for Dogs & Cats:
     Your A-Z Guide to Over 200 Conditions, Herbs,
     Vitamins, and Supplements.* New York: Three Rivers, 2001.
Pitcairn, Richard H., and Susan Hubble Pitcairn. *Dr.
     Pitcairn's New Complete Guide to Natural Health for
     Dogs and Cats.* New York: Rodale Books, 2005.
Schwartz, Cheryl. *Four Paws, Five Directions: A
     Guide to Chinese Medicine for Cats and Dogs.* Berkeley:
     Celestial Arts, 1996.
Stein, Diane. *Natural Healing for Dogs and Cats.* Freedom:
     Crossing, 1993.
Trout, Nick. Tell Me Where It Hurts: A Day of Humor,
     Healing, and Hope in My Life as an Animal Surgeon.
     Broadway, 2009.
The Whole Dog Journal. Web. 09, August 2009.

Websites for Canine Health:

www.assistancedogunitedcampaign.org

www.carecredit.com

Help-A-Pet Veterinary Cost Assistance: *www.help-a-pet.org/*

In Memory of Magic see: *www.imom.org*

Orthodogs' Silver Lining Foundation see: *www.oslf.org*

www.petassure.com/ContactUs.aspx

www.petinsurancereview.com

www.pettech.net (See Dog First Aid information)

www.redcross.org (See Dog First Aid information)

Alternative Healing Resources:

Coates, Margrit. *Hands-On Healing for Pets: The Animal Lover's Essential Guide to Using Healing Energy.* London: Rider, 2004.

Fox, Michael W. *The Healing Touch: The Proven Massage Program for Cats and Dogs.* New York: Newmarket, 1990.

Tellington-Jones, Linda, and Sybil Taylor. *The Tellington Touch: A Revolutionary Natural Method to Train and Care for Your Favorite Animal.* New York: Penguin, 1995.

Alternative Healing Websites:

www.aldaronessences.com/

www.anaflora.com

animalbehaviorassociates.com

www.bachflower.com

www.calmingcollars.com

Turid Rugaas's Website see: *www.canis.no/rugaas/*

www.dogscouts1.com (see relaxation protocol)

www.downeastdognews.com (see identifying and coping with canine stress)

www.healingtouchforanimals.com
Welcome to Chi Institute: Veterinary Acupuncture see:
www.tcvm.com (see Chinese herbal handbook)
www.throughadogsear.com (relaxation music for dogs)
www.thundershirt.com (see ttouch wraps, anxiety wraps, or thundershirts)
www.ttouch.com
http://caninelullabies.com/
www.petalk.org/LaughingDog.html
Nutrition Websites: *www.adogsdreams.tripod.com/*
www.doberdogs.com
www.dogfoodproject.com
www.doggiedietician.com
www.feedmypet.com
www.petdiets.com
www.shirleys-wellness-cafe.com
www.thepossiblecanine.com

Chapter 7: The Golden Years: When to Hang up the Leash
Helping Children Deal With the Loss of their Animal:

Jarrat, Claudia Jewett. *Helping Children Cope with Separation and Loss, Revised Edition.* Harvard Common, 1994.

Kubler-Ross, Elisabeth. *On Children and Death.* New York: Scribner, 1997.

Kubler-Ross, Elisabeth. *On Death and Dying.* New York, N.Y: Simon & Schuster, 1997.

Sife, Wallace. *The Loss of a Pet : New Revised and Expanded Edition.* New York: Howell Book House, 1998.

Wolfelt, Alan. *Helping Children Cope With Grief.* Muncie: Accelerated Development, 1983.

Coping With the Death of Your Dog:

Altomare, Michele Lanci. G*ood-Bye My Friend" Pet Cemeteries, Memorials, and Other Ways to Remember.* New York: BowTie, 2000.

Anderson, Moira K. *Coping With Sorrow on the Loss of Your Pet.* Loveland: Alpine Publications, 1996.

Carmack, Betty J. *Grieving the Death of a Pet.* New York: Augsburg Fortress, 2003.

Milani, Myrna M. *Preparing for the Loss of Your Pet: Saying Goodbye With Love, Dignity, and Pace of Mind.* Rocklin: Prima Pub., 1998.

Tousley, Marty. *Final Farewell: Preparing for & Mourning the Loss of Your Pet.* Phoenix: Our Pals Pub., 1997.

Weaver, Helen. *The Daisy Sutra.* New York: Buddha Rock, 2000.

Coping With the Death of Your Dog Websites & Yahoo Support Group:

www.animalinourhearts.com (see grief support resources)

Association for Pet loss and Bereavement see: *www.aplb.org/*

American veterinary Medical Association see: *www.avma.org*

www.dogtrainingathome.com (see death of a pet)

www.goodgrief.org

www.in-memory-of-pets.com

www.kristi-freeman.com/what_is.html (see: Quality of Life Assessment)

www.petloss.net

www.web.vet.cornell.edu

http://vet.purdue.edu (see pet loss and grief)

Pet Loss Hotline at the College of Veterinary Medicine see: *www.vetmed.wsu.edu/*

Service Dog Bereavement and Grief: *http://groups.yahoo.com/group/grievingaservicedog/*

Index

About the Author

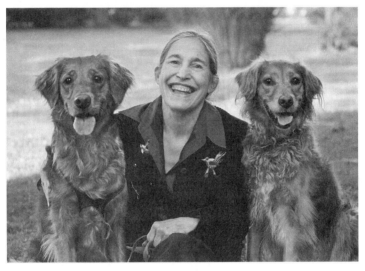

Jane Miller with her two dogs, Ahava (left) and Simcha (right).

Jane Miller, a Licensed Independent Social Worker committed to wholistic modalities of healing, is in practice as a psychotherapist/clinical social worker with her animal-assisted therapy (AAT) dogs. She offers education about and client assessments for Psychiatric Service Dogs (PSDs). Presently, focused on educating others about the legal, ethical, and practical criteria for benefiting from a PSD. Miller has lectured about

PSDs in a variety of settings ranging from national museums to local organizations, schools, and dog-training facilities. She appeared on a PBS program on the healing power of animals and joined world-renowned veterinarian/author Dr. Allen Schoen to present a workshop on the topic of animals as healers at a national conference for medical professionals.

A resident of Northeast Ohio, Miller earned her BA in psychology and biology from Oberlin College, and her MA in Clinical Social Work from Case Western Reserve University. She received the Irene Sogg Gross Award for Humanitarian Services and contributed scholarly essays for professional journals and anthologies in the field of clinical social work. Her professional experience includes serving as a counselor at a battered women's shelter, a group home supervisor for the developmentally disabled, and as a research assistant in microbiology/immunology at Temple University Medical School.

Jane Miller teaches QiGong, Relaxation/Stress Reduction techniques, as well as she is a Reiki practitioner and Energy worker. She appeared on the PBS Series, "Health Visions " presenting an hour long program focused on "QiGong & Healing Energy."

She has been practicing daily meditation and visualization techniques since childhood and has been practicing QiGong daily for 20 years. She practices Reiki on her two therapy dogs daily and teaches her psychotherapy clients stress reduction techniques for their service dogs.

Miller's lifelong passion for healing has emphasized the human-animal connection, culminating in certifications as a Canine Massotherapist and as a Consultant for Therapy and Service Animals by the International Association of Animal Behavior Consultants (IAABC).